VICTORIA WILLS

The Easy Keto Diet Cookbook for Women After 50

Effortless Ketogenic Recipes to Lose Weight Fast, Balance Your Hormones Naturally and Boost Your Health Thanks to Your Stress-Free 28-Day Meal Plan

© Copyright 2020 - All rights reserved.

TABLE OF CONTENTS

Introduction

The keto diet has received great appreciation and praise for its weight loss benefits. This high-fat, low-carbohydrate diet is exceptionally healthy overall. It makes your body burn fat, like a talking machine. Public figures also appreciate it. But the question is, how does Ketosis improve weight loss? Here is a detailed picture of the Ketosis and weight loss process.

Ketosis is considered abnormal by some people. However, it has been approved by many nutritionists and doctors. Many people still disapprove of it. The misconceptions are due to the myths that have spread around the ketogenic diet.

Once your body has no glucose, it will automatically depend on the stored fat. It is also necessary to note that carbohydrates produce glucose, and once you start a low carb diet, you will also be able to lower your glucose levels. Then your body is going to create fuel through fats instead of carbohydrates, that is, glucose.

The process of creating fat through fat is known as Ketosis, and once your body enters this state, it becomes instrumental in burning unwanted fat. Also, since glucose levels are low during the keto diet, your body achieves many other health benefits.

A ketogenic diet is not only beneficial for weight loss, but it also helps positively improve your overall health. Unlike all other diet plans, which focus on reducing calorie intake, Keto emphasizes putting your body in a natural metabolic state, namely Ketosis. The only factor that makes this diet plan questionable is that this nature of metabolism is not much deliberated. With your body making ketones regularly, your body will quickly burn stored fat, leading to tremendous weight loss.

Now the question arises. How does Ketosis affect the human body?

However, this phase does not last more than 2-3 days. This is the time it takes for the human body to enter the ketosis phase. Once you enter it, you will not have any adverse side effects.

Also, you should gradually start reducing your calorie and carbohydrate intake. The most common mistake dietitians make is that they tend to begin eliminating everything from their diet at the same time. This is where the problem arises. The human body will react exceptionally negatively when you limit everything at once. You need to start gradually. Read this guide to learn more about tackling the ketogenic diet after 50.

This diet plan works for both men and women.

This is extremely effective in helping people lose weight and keep it off for a long time.

Weight loss will be followed by constant fatigue and tiredness. Not only will your self-confidence and self-esteem improve, but you'll also be healthier, have more energy, and have fewer mood swings.

It can help both your mind and your body, and the result will be generally positive.

The ketogenic diet can help you start your weight loss journey.

In this e-book, you will learn everything you need to know about maintaining a proper ketogenic diet. This book contains the necessary information on how the diet works, as well as tips for success. Aside from this, you will also find delicious but easy to prepare ketogenic recipes that you would not find difficult to make even if you do not have the luxury of time to do kitchen work.

This book will also give you what you need to flourish with the ketogenic diet—easy cooking, weight loss, and long-term success.

Thanks again for choosing this book, I'd really love to hear your thoughts about it, so make sure to leave a short review on Amazon (with a photo of the book if you enjoy it)

CHAPTER 1:

What is Ketogenic Diet?

You all know that our body needs energy for its functioning, and the energy sources come from carbohydrates, proteins, and fats. Owing to years of conditioning that a low-fat carbohydrate-rich diet is essential for good health, we have become used to depending on glucose (from carbohydrates) to get most of the energy that our body needs. Only when the amount of glucose available for energy generation decreases does our body begin to break down fat for drawing energy to power our cells and organs. This is the express purpose of a ketogenic diet.

The primary aim of a ketogenic diet (called only as of the keto diet) is to convert your body into a fat-burning machine. Such a diet is loaded with benefits and is highly recommended by nutritional experts for the following results:

•Natural appetite control

•Increased mental clarity

•Lowered levels of inflammation in the body system

•Improved stability in blood sugar levels

•Elimination or lower risk of heartburn

•Using natural stored body fat as the fuel source

•Weight loss

The effects listed are just some of the numerous impacts that take place when a person embarks on a ketogenic diet and makes it a point to stick to it. A ketogenic diet consists of meals with low carbohydrates, moderate proteins, and high-fat content. The mechanism works like this: when we drastically reduce the intake of carbohydrates, our body is compelled to convert fat for releasing energy. This process of converting fats instead of carbohydrates to release energy is called Ketosis.

Health Benefits of Keto Diet to Women Above 50

Both low-fat and also low-carb diet plans can be reliable for weight loss, according to the American Association of Retired Persons (AARP). The low-carb diet has some extra health and wellness advantages worth taking into consideration. The researcher also went so far as to recommend that the low-carb diet plan might provide a choice to pain-relieving opioids.

Besides, low-carb diet plans might aid HDL (good) cholesterol and triglyceride degrees much more efficiently than even more carb-heavy diet plans,

according to the Mayo Clinic. Today, low-carb diet plans have taken several popular types, consisting of the keto diet plan, the paleo diet plan, and the Mediterranean diet. While each of these choices includes its nuances, they're all based around lowering carbohydrate intake while raising healthy and balanced fat consumption.

Decreased Thyroid Function

A research study has discovered that a ketogenic diet plan lowers the degree of T3, the body's active thyroid hormonal agent. Unfortunately, this suggests a ketogenic diet might not be optimal for those with preexisting hypothyroidism. Consult with your physician first since you may require thyroid assistance if you have hypothyroidism and also want to continue with a ketogenic diet plan.

Elevated Cortisol

A research study has suggested that a ketogenic diet plan raises the tension hormonal agent cortisol to increase power levels despite reduced carbohydrate availability. It is still debated whether this increase in cortisol is harmless or dangerous. Getting a lot of rest, exercising, and engaging in a routine stress-reduction technique can assist you in keeping your standard tension degrees reduced and decrease the possibility for consistently elevated cortisol.

Nutrient deficiencies: Older grownups often tend to have more significant shortages in essential nutrients like:

Iron: the deficiency can lead to mental fog and also exhaustion

Vitamin B12: deficiency can cause neurological problems like dementia.

Fats: deficiency can lead to troubles with cognition, vitamin, vision, and even skin shortages.

Vitamin D: deficiency can cause cognitive problems in older grownups, raise the danger of cardiovascular disease, and also contribute to cancer cells threat. The top-quality resources of animal protein on the ketogenic diet plan can quickly account for excellent sources of these essential nutrients.

Regulating Blood Sugar

As we've talked about, the connection between low blood sugar and also associated brain circumstances like Alzheimer's disease, mental weakening, and Parkinson's Disease exists. Excess consumption of carbohydrates, mainly from fructose, which is drastically lowered in the ketogenic diet

An absence of nutritional fats and cholesterol-- which are bountiful and also healthy and balanced on the ketogenic diet plan.

Making use of a ketogenic diet to assist in regulating blood sugar levels and improve nourishment might assist not only improve insulin response but also secure against memory issues that frequently transpire with age.

Keto foods provide a high amount of nutrition per calorie. This is crucial because basal metabolic rate (the number of calories needed daily to endure) is less for seniors. Yet, they still need the same quantity of nutrients as younger people.

A person age 50+ will have a much more challenging time residing on junk foods than a teenager or 20+ whose body is still resilient. This makes it also a lot more critical for seniors to eat foods that are disease-fighting and health-supporting. It can necessarily imply the difference between enjoying the golden years to the max or spending them suffering and in pain.

Older women should eat a much better diet plan by avoiding "empty calories" from sugars or nutrient-dense foods such as whole grains and also increasing the amount of healthy, nutrient-rich proteins. Additionally, much of the food chosen by older people (or given up medical facility or clinical settings) often tend to be significantly refined and very poor in nutrients, such as white bread, pasta, prunes, mashed potatoes, puddings, and so on.

It's quite clear that the high-carb diet so commonly pushed by the government is not best for sustaining our senior women and also their lasting health and wellness. A diet plan low in carbs and abundant in animal and plant fats are much better for advertising much better insulin level of sensitivity, and also overall better health and wellness.

Ketosis for Longevity

That being stated, the earlier we can start making changes that support healthy and balanced weight, blood sugar, immunity, and extra, the greater the chance of having less pain and suffering later on in life. Note: We're all growing older, and death is, naturally, unavoidable. People are currently living much longer; however, we're additionally getting sicker by complying with the typical diet plan of the majority. The ketogenic diet can help elders boost their wellness so that they can grow, instead of being ill or hurting during the later years of life.

Because your body turns fat from your diet plan and your inner fat shops into ketones, the keto diet rapidly enhances weight loss. And also, unlike sugar, ketones cannot be stored as fat since they aren't digested similarly.

It's incredible; For decades, you've heard that fat makes you gain weight. Your body has evolved to use fat as a different source of energy. For most of history, people did not eat three meals and snacks all day.

CHAPTER 2:

Why Keto Over 50?

Why Keto for Women?

The health benefits of the Keto diet are not different for men or women, but the speed at which they are reached does differ. As mentioned, women's bodies are a lot other when it comes to the ways that they can burn fats and lose weight. For example, by design, women have at least 10% more body fat than men. Don't be hard on yourself if you notice that it seems like men can lose weight easier — that's because they can! What women have in additional body fat, men typically have the same in muscle mass. This is why men tend to see faster external results because that added muscle mass means that their metabolism rates are higher. That increased metabolism means that fat and energy get burned faster. When you are on Keto, though, the internal change is happening right away.

Your metabolism is unique, but it is also going to be slower than a man's by nature. Since muscle can burn more calories than fat, the weight just seems to fall off of men, giving them the ability to reach the opportunity for muscle growth quickly. As long as you are keeping these realistic bodily factors in mind, you won't be left wondering why it is taking you a little bit longer to start losing weight.

Another unique condition that a woman may experience, but a man may not be polycystic ovary syndrome or polycystic ovary syndrome. A hormonal imbalance that causes cysts to grow. These cysts can cause pain, interfere with normal reproductive function, and, in extreme and dangerous cases, burst. PCOS is ubiquitous among women, affecting up to 10% of the entire female population. Surprisingly, most women are not even aware that they have the condition. Around 70% of women have PCOS, which is undiagnosed. This condition can cause a significant hormonal imbalance, therefore affecting your metabolism. It can also inevitably lead to weight gain, making it even harder to see results while following diet plans.

Menopause is another reality that must be faced by women, especially as we age. Most women begin the process of menopause in their mid-40s. Men do not go through menopause, so they are spared from yet another condition that causes slower metabolism and weight gain. When you start menopause, it is easy to gain weight and lose muscle. Most women, once menopause begins, lose power at a much faster rate, and conversely gain weight, despite dieting and exercise regimens. Keto can, therefore, be the right diet plan for you. Regardless of what your body is doing naturally, via processes like menopause, your internal systems are still going to be making the switch from running on carbs to deriving energy from fats.

Because a Keto diet reduces the amount of sugar you are consuming, it naturally lowers the amount of insulin in your bloodstream. This can have remarkable effects on any existing PCOS and fertility issues, as well as menopausal symptoms and conditions like pre-diabetes and Type 2 diabetes. Once your body adjusts to a Keto diet, you are overcoming the things that are naturally in place that can be preventing you from losing weight and getting healthy. Even if you placed your body on a strict diet, if it isn't getting rid of sugars properly, you likely aren't going to see the same results that you will when you try Keto. This is a big reason why Keto can be so beneficial for women.

As we've deliberated, carbs and sugar can have a significant impact on your hormonal balance. You might not even realize that your hormones are not in the balance until you experience a lifestyle that limits carbs and eliminates sugars. Keto is going to reset this balance for you, keeping your hormones at healthy levels.

Why Keto for 50+?

As we age, we naturally look for ways to hold onto our youth and energy. It's not uncommon to think about things that promote anti-aging. Products and lifestyle changes are advertised everywhere, and they are designed to catch your attention, as you grapple with the reality of what it means to be a 50+-year-old woman in our society. Even if you aren't eating for anti-aging yet, you have likely thought about it in terms of the way you treat your skin and hair, for example.

For instance, indigestion becomes as common as you age. This is because the body cannot break down certain foods like it used to. With all of the additives and fillers, we all become used to putting our bodies through discomfort in an attempt to digest regular meals. You are probably not even aware that you are doing this to your body, but upon trying a Keto diet, you will realize how your digestion will begin to change. You will no longer feel bloated or uncomfortable after you eat. If you notice this as a familiar feeling, you are likely not eating food that is nutritious enough to satisfy your needs and is only resulting in excess calories.

Keto fills you up in all of the ways that you need, allowing your body to digest and metabolize all of the nutrients truly. When you eat your meals, you should not feel the need to overeat to overcompensate for not having enough nutrients. Anything that takes stress off of any system in your body is going to become a form of anti-aging. You will quickly find this benefit once you start your Keto journey, as it is one of the first-reported changes that most participants notice. In addition to a healthier digestive system, you will also experience more regular bathroom usage, with little to none of the problems often associated with age.

While weight loss is one of the more common desires for most 50+ women who start a diet plan, the way that the weight is lost matters. If you have ever shed a lot of weight before, you have probably experienced the adverse effects of sagging or drooping skin that you were left to deal with. Keto rejuvenates the elasticity in your skin. Instead of having to do copious amounts of exercise to firm up your skin, it should already be becoming firmer each day that you are on the Keto diet. This is something that a lot of participants are pleasantly surprised to find out.

Women also commonly report a natural reduction in wrinkles and healthier skin and hair growth, in general. Many women who start the diet report that they notice reverse effects in their aging process. While the skin becomes healthier and more supple, it also becomes firmer. Even if you aren't presently losing weight, you will still be able to appreciate the effects that Keto brings to your skin and face. Because your internal systems are becoming healthier by the day, this tends to show on the outside in a short amount of time. You will also begin to feel healthier. While it is possible to read about the experiences of others, there is nothing like feeling this for yourself when you start Keto.

Everyone, especially women over 50, has day-to-day tasks that are draining and require specific amounts of energy to complete. Aging can, unfortunately, take away from your energy reserve, even if you get enough sleep at night. It limits the way that you have to live your life, and this can become a very frustrating realization. Most diet plans bring about a sluggish feeling that you are simply supposed to get used to, for example. But Keto does the exact opposite. When you change your eating habits to fit the Keto guidelines, you are going to be hit with a boost of energy. Since your body is genuinely getting everything that it needs nutritionally, it will repay you with a sustained energy supply.

Another common complaint about women over 50 is that seemingly overnight, your blood sugar levels are going to be more sensitive than usual. While everyone must keep an eye on these levels, it is especially necessary for those who are in their 50s and beyond. High blood sugar can be an indication that diabetes is on the way, but Keto can become a preventative measure that we've already talked about. Additionally, naturally regulating elevated blood sugar levels also reduces systemic inflammation, which is also common for women over 50. By balancing the immune system, of which inflammation is a part of, everyday aches and pains are reduced. Inflammation can also affect vital organs and is a precursor to cancer. Keto will support your path to an anti-inflammatory lifestyle.

Sugar is never great for us, but it turns out that sugar can become especially dangerous as we age. What is known as a "sugar sag" can occur when you get older because the excess sugar molecules will attach themselves to skin and protein in your body? This doesn't even necessarily happen because you are overeating sugar. Average levels of sugar intake can also lead to this sagging as the sugar weakens the strength of your proteins that are supposed to hold you together. With sagging comes even more wrinkles and arterial stiffening.

If you have any anti-aging concerns, the Keto diet will likely be able to address your worries. It is a diet that works extremely hard while allowing you a relatively direct and straightforward guideline to follow in return. While your motivation is necessary to form a successful relationship with Keto, you will not have to worry about doing something "wrong" or accidentally breaking out of your diet. Once you know how to give up sugary foods and drinks while making sure you consume the right amount of carbs, you will be able to find your success while on a diet.

As a woman over 50, you'll find that you will feel better, healthier, and younger, by implementing the simple steps that will tune your body into processing excess fats for energy. You'll build muscle, lose fat, and look and feel younger. As we've touched on, a Keto diet helps balance your hormones, reversing and eliminating many common menopausal signs and symptoms.

CHAPTER 3:

Types of Keto Diet

There are several types of Ketogenic diet that you could adapt and maintain. These include;

The Standard Ketogenic Diet (SKD):
In simple terms, this is a very low-carb diet accompanied by high-fats and moderate protein that is consumed by human beings. It consists of 70% to 75% fats, 20% protein and about 5% to 10% carbs. This translates to about 20 – 45 grams of carbohydrates, 40 – 65 grams of proteins, but no set limits for fats, which makes up for large parts of the diet. This is because fats are what provide the calories which constitute energy and make the diet a successful Ketogenic diet. Additionally, there is no limit to the fats because different human beings have different energy requirements. The Standard Ketogenic Diet is successful in assisting people in losing weight, improving the body's glucose as well as improving heart health.

Targeted Ketogenic Diet (Tkd)
This type of Ketogenic Diet focuses its attention on the addition of carbs during workout sessions only. This type of Ketogenic diet is almost similar to the Standard Ketogenic Diet except for the fact that carbohydrates are all but consumed during workout sessions. This type of diet is solely based on the idea that the body will effectively and efficiently process carbohydrates consumed before or during a workout session. This is because the diet assumes that the muscles would be bound to demand more energy, which would be provided by the carbohydrates consumed and be processed quickly since the body is in an active state. This diet, in simpler terms, is a diet caught up between the Cyclical Ketogenic diet and the Standard Ketogenic Diet, which allows room for consumption of carbohydrates on the days that you would decide to work out only.

High-Protein Ketogenic Diet
This type of Ketogenic Diet advocates for more protein compared to the Standard Ketogenic Diet. This diet consists of 35% protein, 60% fats, and 5% carbs, unlike the Standard Ketogenic Diet. Research has dramatically suggested that this diet would be useful for you if you are attempting to lose weight. However, unlike other types of the Ketogenic diet, no research has been dedicated to showing if there are any side effects of adapting to the diet for elongated periods.

Recurring Ketogenic Diet (RKD)
This kind of Ketogenic Diet focuses on higher-carb re-feeds, for instance, 5 Ketogenic days and two high-carb days, and this cycle is repeated. This diet is also known as the carb backloading. It is often intended for athletes because the diet allows their bodies to recover the glycogen lost as a result of workouts or intense sporting activities.

Very Low Carbs Ketogenic Diet (VLCKD)
As stated prior, a Ketogenic diet will most likely consist of very low carbs; thus, this diet often refers to the characteristics of the Standard Ketogenic Diet.

The Well Formulated Ketogenic Diet:

this term is as a result of one of the leading researchers into the Ketogenic diet, Steve Phinney. As the name suggests, this diet has its fats, carbohydrates, and proteins well-formulated, and that it meets the standards of a Ketogenic diet. This diet is also similar to the Standard Ketogenic Diet, and this means that it creates room for your body to undergo Ketosis effectively.

The Mct Ketogenic Diet:

The diet is also related to the Standard Ketogenic Diet only that it derives most of its fats from medium-chain triglycerides (MCTs). This diet will often use coconut oil, which has high levels of MCTs. This diet has been reported to efficiently treat epilepsy because of its concept that MCTs give your body enough room to consume carbohydrates as well as proteins and still maintain your body's Ketosis. This is a result of MCTs providing more ketones per gram in fat, contrary to the long-chain triglycerides, which are more common in the average dietary fats. However, MCTs could lead to diarrhea as well as stomach upsets if this diet is consumed in large quantities on its own. To handle, it is wise to prepare a meal with a balance of both MCTs and fats with no MCTs. There is no evidence to prove that this diet could as well have benefits in your attempt to losing weight or if the diet could regulate your body's blood sugar.

The Calorie Restricted Ketogenic Diet

This is also related to the Standard Ketogenic Diet except that its calories are only limited to a given amount. Research has proven that Ketogenic diets could be successful whether the consumption of calories is restricted or not. The reason behind this is that the effect of consuming fats and your body being in Ketosis is a way in itself that prevents you from over-eating or eating beyond your limits.

There are numerous Ketogenic diets, but the Standard Ketogenic Diet and the High-Protein Ketogenic Diets are the most studied and most recommended for health issues. The Repeated (cyclical) and Targeted Ketogenic diets remain mostly practiced by athletes and bodybuilders and are more advanced than the Standard Ketogenic Diet and the High-Protein Ketogenic Diet. Visit and consult your local physician before opting to settle on any of the types of Ketogenic diets.

CHAPTER 4:

How Does the Ketogenic Diet Work?

The time has come for you to get the answer to the question that has been lingering in your mind from the time you heard about the keto diet; 'how does a keto diet work?'

Here is how.

The power behind the Ketogenic diet's ability to help you lose weight and have better health comes from a straightforward action that the diet initiates in your body once you start following it. This simple action is how the keto diet changes your metabolism from burning carbohydrates for energy to burning fats.

What does that have to do with weight loss and better health?

Let me break it down for you.

• Burning carbohydrate for energy

Most of the food we eat follow the food pyramid recommended by the USDA a few decades ago. The pyramid puts carbohydrates at the bottom of the pyramid and fats at the top of the pyramid, which essentially means that carbohydrates form the bulk of the foods we eat, as shown below:

What many of us don't know is that when you consume a diet that is high in carbohydrates, two things naturally happen.

• One, your body takes the just consumed carbohydrates and converts it into glucose, which is the easiest molecule that your body can convert to use as energy (glucose is your body's primary source of life, as it gets chosen over any other energy source in your body).

• Secondly, your body produces insulin for the sole purpose of it moving the glucose from your bloodstream into your cells where it can be used as energy.

There is more that goes unnoticed though:

Since your body gets its energy from glucose (which is mostly in massive amounts because we eat lots of high carb food 3-6 times a day), it doesn't need any other source of energy. Many are the times when glucose is in excess, something that prompts the body to convert dietary glucose into glycogen to be stored in the liver and muscle cells. What this simple explanation means is that with a high carb diet, your body is essentially in what we refer to as a fat-storing mode. It stores this excess fat so that it can use it when starved from its primary source of energy; glucose. Unfortunately, since we don't give ourselves enough breaks from food, we end up being in this constant fat-storing mode that ultimately causes weight gain.

• Burning fats for energy

As you now know, the Ketogenic diet is a low carb, high fat, and moderate protein diet. So, when you start following a Ketogenic diet, what typically happens is, your intake of carbohydrates is kept at a low. In other words, it inverts the USDA food pyramid I mentioned earlier, something that literally 'inverts/reverses' the effects of a high carb diet.

How exactly does it do that?

Well, when you limit your carb intake much, you starve the body of its primary source of energy, something that initiates the process that the body has always been preparing for through its energy storage processes. More specifically, the body starts by metabolizing glycogen with the help of glucagon hormone (the process takes place in the liver). And with support from the human growth hormone, cortisol, and catecholamines (norepinephrine to be more specific), the body starts releasing fatty acids for use as energy in different body parts. But since fatty acids cannot be used by every cell in the body, the body is also forced to transport some of the fatty acids to the liver where they are broken down in a series of metabolic processes known as Ketosis to produce three ketone bodies. Therefore, Ketosis is a natural process that your body activates when your energy intake is low to help you to survive. The three ketones that are formed when fatty acids are converted are:

- Acetone.

- Beta-hydroxybutyric acid (BHB)

- Acetoacetate (AcAc)

Many of your body cells (including the brain cells) can use BHB for energy, as it is water-soluble, something that makes it very much like glucose in that it can cross the blood-brain barrier. The more ketones the body cells use for energy, the more fat you are burning, and ultimately, the more weight you stand to gain. This essentially means a Ketogenic diet makes your body a fat-burning machine, as it relies primarily on fats (both dietary and stored body fat – though you want to get your body to burn as much of the stored boy fat as possible).

Ketosis helps you get rid of excessive fats in your body, which not only reduces your weight in a big way but also betters your health by protecting you from various diseases, as you will see.

To attain Ketosis, you know that your intake of fats should be high, intake of carbs low, and intake of proteins moderate. But what exactly does high, low, and moderate translate to in calorie terms? In simpler terms, in what ratios should you take carbs, fats, and proteins? This gives rise to several types/approaches/schools of thought regarding the rates:

Who invented this diet?

The ketogenic diet traces its roots to the treatment of epilepsy. Surprisingly this goes all the way back to 500 BC when ancient Greeks observed that fasting or eating a ketogenic diet helped reduce epileptic seizures. In modern times, the ketogenic diet was reintroduced in the practice of medicine to treat children with epilepsy.

What is Ketosis?

Ketosis is a metabolic state where the body is efficiently using fat for energy. In a regular diet, carbohydrates produce glucose, which is used to provide power. Glucose is stored in the body in fat cells that travel via the bloodstream. People gain weight when there is fatter stored than being used as energy.

Glucose is formed through the consumption of sugar and starch—namely carbohydrates. The sugars may be in the form of natural sugars from fruit or milk, or they may be formed from processed sugar. Starches like pasta, rice, or starchy vegetables like potatoes and corn form glucose as well. The body breaks down the sugars from these foods into glucose. Glucose and insulin combined to help to carry glucose into the bloodstream so the body can use glucose as energy. The glucose that is not used is stored in the liver and muscles.

For the body to supply ketones for use as fuel, the body must use up all the reserves of glucose. A very low carb diet, the production of ketones what her to feel the body and brain.

Ketones are produced from the liver when there is not enough glucose in the body to provide energy. When insulin levels are low, and there is not enough glucose or sugar in the bloodstream, fat is released from fat cells and travels in the blood to the liver. The liver processes the fat into ketones. Ketones are released into the bloodstream to provide fuel for the body and increase the body's metabolism. Ketones are formed under conditions of starvation, fasting, or a diet low in carbohydrates.

CHAPTER 5:

How the Keto Diet Affects 50 Old Women

Women who are looking for a quick and effective way to shed excess weight, get high blood sugar levels under control, reduce overall inflammations, and improve physical and mental energy will do their best by following a ketogenic diet plan. But there are special considerations women must take into account when they are beginning the keto diet.

All women know it is much more difficult for women to lose weight than it is for men to lose weight. A woman will live on a starvation level diet and exercise like a triathlete and only lose five pounds. A man will stop putting dressing on his salad and will lose twenty pounds. It just is not fair. But we have the fact that we are women to blame. Women naturally have more standing between them and weight loss than men do.

The mere fact that we are women is the largest single contributor to the reason we find it difficult to lose weight. Since our bodies always think they need to be prepared for the possibility of pregnant women will naturally have more body fat and less mass in our muscles than men will. So, because we are women, we will always lose weight more slowly than men will.

Being in menopause will also cause women to add more pounds to their bodies, especially in the lower half of the body. After menopause, a woman's metabolism naturally slows down. Your hormone levels will decrease. These two factors alone will cause weight gain in the post-menopausal woman.

Women are a direct product of their hormones. Men also have hormones but not the ones like we have that regulate every function in our bodies. And the hormones in women will fluctuate around their everyday habits like lack of sleep, poor eating habits, and menstrual cycles. These hormones cause women to crave sweets around the time their periods occur. These cravings will wreck any diet plan. Staying true to the keto plan is challenging at this time because of the intense desire for sweets and carbs. Also, having your period will often make you feel and look bloated because of the water your body holds onto during this time. And they have cramps make you more likely to reach for a bag of cookies than a plate of steak and salad.

Because we are women, we may experience challenges on the keto diet that men will not face because they are men. One of these challenges is having a weight loss plateau or even experiencing weight gain. If this happens, you will want to increase your consumption of good fats like ghee, butter, eggs, coconut oil, beef, avocados, and olive oil. Any food that is cooked or prepared using oil must be prepared in olive oil or avocado oil.

You can also use MCT oil. MCT stands for medium-chain triglycerides. MCT can help with many body functions, from weight loss to improved brain function. MCTs are mostly missing from the typical American diet because we have been told that saturated fats are harmful to the body, and as a group they are. But certain saturated fats, like MCTs, are beneficial to the body, especially when they come from the right foods like beef or coconut oil.

Many women on a keto diet will struggle with imbalances in their hormones. On the keto diet, you do not rely on lowered calories to lose weight but on foods' effect on your hormones. So, when women begin the keto diet any issues, they are already having with their hormones will be brought to attention and may cause the woman to give up before she starts. Always remember that the keto diet is responsible for cleansing the system first so that the body can quickly respond to the beautiful effects a keto diet has to offer.

Do not try to work toward the lean body that many men sport. It is best for an overall function that women stay at twenty-two to twenty-six percent body fat. Our hormones will function best in this range, and we can't possibly work without our hormones. Women who are very lean, like gymnasts and extreme athletes, will find their hormones no longer function or function at a less than optimal rate. And remember that ideal weight may not be the right weight for you. Many women find that they perform their best when they are at their happy weight. If you find yourself fighting with yourself to lose the last few pounds you think you need to lose to have the perfect body, then it may not be worth it. The struggle will affect your hormone function. Carefully observing the keto diet will allow time for your hormones to stabilize and regulate themselves back to their pre-obesity normal function.

Like any other diet plan, the keto diet will work better if you are active. Regular exercise will allow the body to strengthen and tone muscles and will help to work off excess fat reserves. But training requires energy to accomplish. If you restrict your carb intake too much, you might not have the energy needed to be physically able to make it through the day and still be able to maintain an exercise routine.

As a woman, you know that sometimes your emotions get the better of you. This is true with your body, as you well know, and can be a significant reason why women find it extremely difficult at times to lose weight the way they want to lose weight. We have been led to believe that not only can we do it all but that we must do it all. This gives many women extreme levels of pressure and can cause them to engage in emotional eating. Some women might have lowered feelings of self-worth and may not feel they are entitled to the benefits of the keto diet, and turning to food relieves the feelings of inadequacy that we try to hide from the world.

When you engage in the same activity for an extended period, it becomes a habit. When you reach for the bag of potato chips or the tub of ice cream whenever you are angry, upset, or depressed, then your brain will eventually tell you to reach for food whenever you feel an emotion that you don't want to deal with. Food acts as a security blanket against the world outside. It may be necessary to address any extreme emotional issues you are having before you begin the keto diet, so that you are better assured of success.

The actual act of staying on the keto diet can be very challenging for some women. Many women see beginning a new diet to lose weight as a punishment for being overweight. It may be worthwhile for you to work at changing the settings of your mind if you are feeling this way. You may need to remind yourself daily that the keto diet is not a punishment but a blessing for your body. Tell yourself that you do not deny yourself certain foods because you can't eat them, but because you do not like the way those foods make your body feel. Don't watch other people eating their high carb diet and pity yourself. Instead, feel sorry for the people who have trapped themselves in a high-calorie diet and are not experiencing the benefits that you are experiencing.

And for the first thirty days, cut out all sweeteners, even the non-sugar ones that are allowed on the keto diet. While they may make food taste better, they also remind your brain that it needs sweet foods when it doesn't. Cutting them out for at least thirty days will break the cycle that your body has fallen into and will cut the cravings for sweets in your diet.

Women can be successful on the keto diet if they are prepared to follow a few simple adjustments that will make the diet look differently than your male partner might be eating, but that will make you successful in the long run.

The third benefit from eating more fat, and perhaps the most important, is the psychological boost you will get from seeing that you can eat more fat and still lose weight and feel good. It will also reset your mindset that you formerly might have held against fat. For so long, we have been told that low fat is the only way to lose weight. But an absence of dietary fat will lead to overeating and binge eating out of a feeling of deprivation. When you begin the diet by allowing yourself to eat a lot, or too much in your mind, fat, then you swing the pendulum around to the other side of the fat scale where it properly belongs. You teach yourself that fat can be right for you. Increasing the extra intake of fats should not last beyond the second week of the diet. Your body will improve its ability to create and burn ketones and body fat, and then you will begin using your body fat for fuel, and you can begin to lower your reliance on dietary fat a little bit so that you will start to lose weight.

The keto diet is naturally lower in calories if you follow the recommended levels of food intake. It is not necessary to try to restrict your intake of calories even further. All you need to do is to eat only until you are full and not one bite more. Besides losing weight, the keto diet aims to retrain your body on how to work correctly. You will need to learn to trust your body and the signals it sends out to be able to readjust to a proper way of eating.

CHAPTER 6:

Entering the State of Ketosis to Lose Weight and Stay Healthy

Ketogenic Vs. Low Carb

Keto and low carbohydrate diets are similar in many ways. On a ketogenic diet, the body moves to a ketosis state, and ketones ultimately power the brain. These are produced in the liver when the intake of carbohydrates is minimal. Low carbohydrate diets may entail various things for different people. Low-carb diets reduce your overall carbohydrate consumption.

For regular low-carb diets, brain habits are still mostly glucose-dependent, although they may consume higher ketones than standard diets. To accomplish this, you'd have to follow low-carb, low-calorie, and an active lifestyle. The amount of carbohydrate you eat depends on the type of diet you consume.

Low carb is reduced in your carb intake. Mentions can vary enormously depending on the number of total carbs consumed per day. People have different views and follow additional rules, from 0 to 100 grams of net carbs. Though a ketogenic diet has low carbohydrates, it also has significantly low protein levels. The overall increase in blood levels of ketones is significant.

What Is Ketosis?

When you reduce the intake of carbs over a while, the body can begin to break down body fat for energy for daily tasks. This is a natural occurrence called Ketosis that the body undergoes to help us survive while food intake is small. We create ketones during this process, produced from the breakdown of fats in the liver. Once ketones are processed into energy, they are a byproduct of fatty acids. Blood ketone bodies also increase substantially to higher than normal levels. Mind, muscle, and all tissue that includes mitochondria utilize ketones. With practice, you'll soon learn how to understand ketosis signs.

An adequately controlled ketogenic diet has the function of pushing your body into the metabolic state to consume fats as energy, not by depriving the body of calories but by eliminating sugars. The bodies are outstandingly resilient to what you place in them. Taking keto nutrients such as keto OS can improve cell regeneration, strength, and lifespan. If an excess of fats is available, and carbs are eliminated, ketones can continue to burn as the primary source of energy.

Can A Keto Diet Help You Lose Weight?

There are different ways that a ketogenic diet will help a person shed excess fat in their body to meet their target weight. Scientists are still doing thorough research to understand just how this whole process works and how precisely the condition of Ketosis helps an individual in terms of losing their excess weight.

With improved satiety and dieting plans, binge eating is something that can usually be avoided effectively. If you don't feel hungry between the main meals of the day, there's little need for a bag of potato chips or an energy bar.

CHAPTER 7:

Signs and Symptoms, You're in Ketosis

As you practice the ketogenic diet further, you will be able to tell you are in Ketosis through the signs and symptoms you are going to experience. Remember that you will now be providing your body with a new fuel source. It is going to take a little bit of time to adapt your body to this change. Below, you will find the most common symptoms of Ketosis to tell if you are following the diet correctly.

Bad Breath

I know, a great introduction to the ketogenic diet, but bad breath is one of the most reported symptoms for individuals who have reached full Ketosis. The good news is that this is a widespread side effect for individuals who follow a low-carb diet. Some have described the scent as a "fruit" smell.

Elevated ketone levels in your body cause this scent. The smell is the acetone that exits your body through breath and urine. And while this symptom is less than ideal for your friends and family, it is an excellent sign that you are following your diet correctly! To solve this issue, you will want to brush your teeth a few times a day or find a sugar-free gum to chew on.

Increased Ketones in Blood, Urine, or Breath

As mentioned earlier, you will want to find a method of testing ketones in your body. One of the best ways to do this is to test your blood ketone levels using a meter. When you do this, the meter will be able to measure the amount of BHB in your blood, one of the primary ketones that will be present in your bloodstream. If you are in true Ketosis, your blood ketones should be anywhere from .5-3.0 mmol/L.

Weight Loss

When you first begin the ketogenic diet, weight loss can happen almost immediately. Some have reported that weight loss has even occurred in the first week! If this happens, the weight loss is most likely coming from the water and carbs that have been stored in your body. After the initial drop in weight, you should expect to lose body fat consistently. It will be up to you to stick to the diet to keep the weight loss up!

Decreased Appetite

Another common symptom of the ketogenic diet is appetite suppression. Many individuals have reported that while following this diet, they aren't as hungry as they used to be. Potentially, this could be due to the increased protein intake and alterations to the hunger hormones through Ketosis. Either way, a decreased appetite means increased weight loss. It is a win-win situation for anyone following the ketogenic diet.

Increased Energy

When your body enters Ketosis, you will probably experience a new boost of energy that you didn't even know you had in you! Of course, increased energy and focus are a long-term effect of the diet. When you first start, you will most likely experience symptoms such as tiredness and brain fog. Fret not, as this is to be expected as your body adapts to a new fuel source.

The good news is that once you are in Ketosis, your brain is going to start burning these ketones instead of glucose. This is a very potent fuel for your mind, which is why followers of this diet have reported improved brain function and clarity.

Fatigue

As mentioned earlier, more than likely, you will experience some fatigue if you are just getting started on the ketogenic diet. On top of exhaustion, you may feel overall weak, which is a pretty common side effect of the ketogenic diet. As you probably realize, the switch to running on ketones isn't going to happen overnight. Instead, you should expect these symptoms to subside anywhere from seven to thirty days. To help combat the fatigue, consider taking an electrolyte supplement.

Digestive Issues

Another common symptom of starting this diet is experiencing digestive issues. When you make such a drastic change to your diet, it involves changing the types of foods you eat daily. When this happens, digestive problems like diarrhea and constipation are to be expected. While these symptoms will subside, you may want to take note of which foods you feel are causing these issues...

The Keto Flu and How to Survive

The ketogenic diet seems to be reasonably infamous for the keto flu. As your body begins to adapt to the new fuel source, it can genuinely feel like the flu. You may experience several symptoms such as dizziness, stomach pains, fatigue, and overall tiredness. For many beginners, this is the end of their attempt at the ketogenic diet.

You see, the keto flu is not caused by Ketosis or ketogenesis. The keto flu is caused by your body and its reaction to carbohydrate restriction! For many, this is the hardest part of following the ketogenic diet, but if you can make it through (I promise you can), incredible benefits are waiting on the other side.

The question here is, why is it so hard for the body to give up carbohydrates? You can look at carbs as your body's first love. Carbohydrates have provided free energy for your body up until this point. But, those carbohydrates are causing harm by increasing the risk of obesity, heart disease, and even diabetes. As you begin to break up with carbohydrates, it's going to be difficult at first.

While the adaption period is going to be difficult, through a proper diet of protein and fat, your body will begin to produce ketones and begin to feel so much better. But in the meantime, your body is going to have to adapt through different changes not just on a cellular level but also on a hormonal level. So, what can you expect when first starting? Below, you will find some of the signs and symptoms you are to expect in the first week or so of being the ketogenic diet.

Symptoms of the Keto Flu

While the keto flu may feel like the end of the world to some people, the good news is that it only lasts about a week for most people. You can expect these symptoms to begin around a day or two after you cut carbs from your diet. You can expect the following:

•Insomnia

•Confusion

•Muscle Soreness

•Nausea

•Stomach Pains

•Cramping

•Poor Concentration

•Irritability

•Inability to Focus

•Brain Fog

•Sugar Cravings

•Dizziness

Don't worry, though, you are likely experiencing only a few of these symptoms. For the lucky few, you may not even have gotten over the keto flu, but you better be prepared for the worst, just in case! You see, the keto flu affects everyone differently!

The main culprit for the keto flu will be your body's metabolic flexibility. This flexibility refers to its ability to adapt to the new availability and source of fuel. You may be wondering, can I be more flexible? The answer is yes, and no.

Your metabolic flexibility involves two things: genetics and lifestyle. If you look at it genetically, some people are born with less metabolic flexibility. For these unfortunate individuals, this means that it will be more challenging to adapt to the ketogenic diet, although not impossible.

If you want to be more flexible throughout your lifestyle, take a look at what you eat before starting the ketogenic diet. If your diet consists of a lot of processed foods and refined sugar, you are much more likely to experience the symptoms of a ketogenic diet.

Why Is This Happening to Me?

By having a deeper understanding of why keto flu occurs first, you will be able to understand better how to alleviate severe symptoms. Blessed with metabolic flexibility or not, your body undergoes drastic changes when you reduce carbohydrates. We've narrowed you down to some of the top culprits that can cause your symptoms.

Sodium and Water

First up, we have the fact that both water and sodium are now being flushed out of your system (bye water weight!). As you begin to restrict the number of carbohydrates in your diet, this is going to trigger the insulin release. As this insulin starts to tell your cells that there is an excess amount of energy in the body, this is going to begin your kidneys to hold onto water and sodium. On the ketogenic diet, these levels are going to drop, and the sodium will be released from your body, taking all of the water with it. Typically, you can expect up to ten pounds of water weight lost in the first five days of your diet!

While seeing the number on your scale drop is going to be exciting, you will feel like garbage if this isn't taken care of properly. On top of the sodium and water leaving your body, the glycogen and fluid levels are going to be released as well. Through this process, the water loss could lead to symptoms such as headaches, dizziness, cramping, nausea, and gastrointestinal issues. This is why drinking the proper amount of water is going to be vital. You must replenish those minerals and fluids in your body.

Increased Cortisol Levels

As you begin the ketogenic diet, you will be triggering a response in your body, telling it that you are starving. While this is far from the truth, your body, who isn't used to living without carbohydrates, is going to release the stress hormone known as cortisol.

Once you become adapted to the ketones, these cortisol levels should balance out. Generally, this process takes a few weeks, depending on several different factors, including your diet, lifestyle, and that metabolic flexibility.

CHAPTER 8:

The Science Behind It

The idea behind most diets remains the same. One needs to reduce the amount of carbs intake in a day, and the weight should fall. The problem is that most diets require you to stop eating or skip meals to bring the carb level down. For a very long time, I had wondered if there was any other way to address this issue.

Indeed, the idea of losing weight is appealing. It is a motivator that pushes us to stop eating and force our body to start converting stored fats into fuel to burn. Sounds good, but the hunger that comes in is a killer.

The catch behind cutting down on carbs is simple. It makes your body run low on glucose. When that happens, the state of Ketosis is in effect. This is where ketones come to the rescue as your body's natural fuel backup. Here's a little fact: we only ever enter into the state of Ketosis if we starve ourselves for a few days, not just overnight or by skipping a meal. That, then, is quite a challenging prospect.

In Keto, things work a little differently, and fortunately a little more friendly. The principle remains the same, you force your body to switch the ketosis mode on, but instead of starving yourself for food, you just cut down the amount of carbs while continuing to consume other nutrients. Slice it any way you like, but this is genuinely more interesting and easier to do.

By removing all sorts of carbs, including but not limited to complex carbs, starches, and refined carbs, we will force our body to lose glucose and be left with no other source to acquire more. This will then switch our body into Ketosis to allow ketones to make their way to the brain and resume normal functions. Our brain requires either glucose or ketones to function, and through Ketosis, it gets the necessary supply.

What follows afterward is a continuous process of our body breaking down fats into ketones regardless of how much protein or fat you consume. The result is a satisfying hunger and weight loss that changes everything for you; a feat many diets cannot deliver.

People have been criticized for how easy this diet can be and how it can produce great results. Ketogenic diets are for almost everyone who suffers from weight problems and cannot lose the extra pounds. By choosing your food carefully and monitoring your keto intake, you should be able to see results fairly quickly.

It goes without saying that for a weight loss solution, Keto seems like a perfect candidate. Not only do you not have to stop eating, but you can enjoy delicious meals while losing weight through techniques that would otherwise require starving yourself. Aside from these facts, most keto recipes are straightforward to cook, and most of them taste just as delicious. This means you don't have to rely on bitter-tasting drinks, strange food, or a lack of it.

Why Is It Important for People Over 50?

Now comes the exciting part. I am sure you have been wondering how it will help you, a person who is 50 years or more in age, and why is it so important, right? Do not worry as I shall provide you with an answer that satisfies both questions.

A few minutes ago, we read how keto diet pushes our body into ketosis, a state where ketones take over the role of glucose. That may sound good for younger people than you, but the fact is that it is a better fit for someone your age. Why I hear you ask?

As you grow in age, the body's natural fat-burning ability reduces. When that happens, your body stops receiving a healthy dose of nutrients properly, which is why you will develop diseases and ailments. With the keto diet, you are pushing the body into Ketosis and bypassing the need to worry about your body's ability to burn fat. Once in Ketosis, your body will now burn fat forcefully for survival.

Once more, your system will now start to regain strength. An even better aspect that follows is your insulin level because it drops. If you are someone diagnosed with diseases such as type 2 diabetes and others, the drop in insulin might even reverse the effects and eliminate the infections from your body altogether.

There are studies underway, and most of them suggest that the keto diet is far more beneficial to those above 50 than it is for those under this age bracket. That is a staggering number for a diet plan that has only been around a few years.

It is also important to highlight that as we get older, we start losing more than just the ability to burn fat. During this phase of our life, once we hit around 50 years of age, we come across various obstacles, some chronic in nature, which transpire only because our body is no longer able to function at rates like it did when we were young. Ketogenic diets help us regain that edge and feel energized from within.

There are hundreds of thousands of stories, all pointing out how this revolutionary diet is especially helpful for older adults and the elderly. It is, therefore, a no-brainer for people above 50 who have spent ages trying to search for a healthy lifestyle choice of diet. With such a high success rate, there is no harm in trying, right?

Before the keto phenomenon, there was the Atkins diet. The Atkins diet was also a low carb diet, just like its keto counterpart. This form of diet also became a massive hit with the masses. However, unlike Keto, the Atkins diet provided weight loss while putting a person through constant hunger. Keto, on the other hand, takes away that element, and it does that using Ketosis.

Constant exposure to Ketosis reduces appetite, hence taking away the biggest hurdle in most diets. The Atkins diet failed to address that front, which is why it was more of a hit and miss. However, credit where it is due, the Atkins diet did garner quite a bit of fame. However, since the inception of Keto, things have changed dramatically.

A study was conducted where 34 overweight adults were monitored and observed for 12 months. All of them were put on keto diets. The result showed that participants had lower HgbA1c (hemoglobin A1c) levels, experienced significant weight loss, and were more likely to discontinue their medications for diabetes altogether.

All in all, the keto diet is shaping up to be quite a promising candidate for older adults. Not only will this diet allow us to lead a healthier lifestyle, but it will also curb our ailments and ensure high energy around the clock. That is quite the resume for a diet and one that now seems too attractive to pass up. This is the point where I made up my mind and decided to give the keto diet a go, and I recommend the same to you.

.

Keto has been producing results that have attracted the top minds and researchers for a reasonably long time. Considering the unique nature of this lifestyle of eating, the results have been somewhat encouraging.

"Great! How do I start?"

Not so fast. While the keto diet is simple, there are a few things I should point out, which you should know. Some of these might even change your mind about the entire keto diet plan, but if you are determined for a healthy lifestyle and a fit body, I assure you these should not be of much trouble.

Preparing Yourself for Keto

When entering the world of Keto, quite a few of us just pick up a recipe on the internet and start cooking things accordingly. While that is good, we do tend to search for any specifics which we should know of, such as what would happen if I replace nuts with something else? Is oatmeal a part of the keto diet? What is Keto approved food items? Are there any risks involved?

Here is more information on such questions:

Keto is an extremely strict food diet where you can only eat things that can be described as Keto that are worth it.

Keto is a whole new way of life. This means that your body will undergo some changes. While most of these will be fine, some can cause problems like the keto flu. Most of the people I know, including myself, have experienced this "flu" with flu-like symptoms. Only after some research did I realize it was natural. Keto flu isn't exactly a cause for concern, but it's best to be mentally prepared for it.

You will need to practice your culinary skills, as the ketogenic diet strongly encourages processed foods that are high in carbohydrates.

If you're not interested in the idea of protein and fat intake, you might want to reconsider, as these are the two main areas Keto focuses on.

Apart from this, there are some mistakes that people tend to make when starting their journey. Some of the most common mistakes are:

Not knowing keto foods correctly - Just because something looks like a keto-friendly item doesn't mean it's Keto approved. Always consult a food guide to check if the thing you are interested in is part of the "good food" in Keto.

Maintain the same level of fat intake at all times - This often leads to results that appear at first and then disappear. You need to continually adjust your diet and monitor your protein and fat intake.

Drink bulletproof coffee when you really shouldn't - this coffee contains a mixture of coconut oil and butter in coffee. While it's a perfect way to keep hunger at bay, it does raise bad cholesterol. If you are someone who has been advised to maintain cholesterol levels and avoid eating similar foods, save it to a minimum.

Just a little break to ask you something that means a lot for me: Are you enjoying this book? If so, I'd be really happy if you could leave a short review on Amazon. I'm so curious to know your opinion! Don't forget to add a photo of the book if you can, thank you.

CHAPTER 9:

Benefits of Keto for Seniors After 50

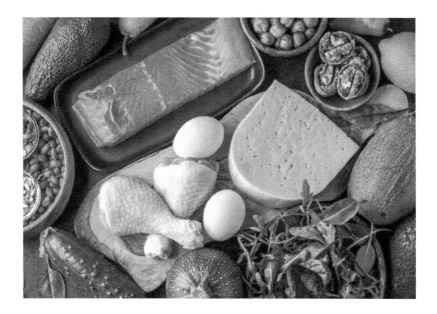

There are a lot of benefits to starting a ketogenic diet, be it in terms of weight, experience or to improve your health!

Effective in Fighting Epilepsy

The primary goal of this diet, introduced in Antiquity, was to fight against epilepsy. The ketones may affect anti-convulsion, but to date, it is not possible to say why they have this effect on the body.

Without going too far into the scientific part, ketone bodies would have an impact on the concentrations of glutamate and GABA (Gamma-Amino Butyric Acid). Glutamate is the main excitatory neuro-mediator of the central nervous system, and GABA, the main inhibitory neuro-mediator. This would explain why the ketogenic diet has such essential effects on people with epilepsy. But I don't want to lose you with my scientific explanations, you can do your research if the subject interests you.

Effective in Weight Loss

Your body's source of energy in the ketogenic diet is fat, either from food or stored by your body. This, therefore, has advantages: the level of insulin, a hormone that stores fat, drops very significantly, this means that your body will become more efficient at burning fat.

Effective in Type I or Type II Diabetes

Diabetes results in a problem in the metabolism of carbohydrates. The diet is, therefore, naturally a place to relieve the signs and symptoms in a person with diabetes, whether for a type I or type II diabetes. Whether the problem is a defect in insulin production or insulin resistance, the ketogenic diet will make it possible to get around the problem.

When you are Keto-adapted, your blood sugar drops sharply because you only eat foods low in carbohydrates. The ketogenic diet can, therefore, allow you to control your blood sugar, which can be very useful in managing your diabetes. The ketogenic diet will allow you to reduce your insulin levels to healthy and stable values.

Effective in People with Alzheimer's

Excuse me in advance, but in this part, we will tackle a scientific "hair" side to explain the benefits of the ketogenic diet in the treatment of Alzheimer's disease.

In addition to all this, the ketogenic diet would have a role in protecting against oxidative stress, and therefore would be preventive and effective against cell death. This would, therefore, limit brain degeneration.

Improves Concentration

The ketones are an excellent source of fuel for the brain. As you decrease your carbohydrate intake, you avoid blood sugar spikes, which often appear after meals. This allows your body to prevent focusing on eliminating carbohydrates and concentrate on the activity you are doing.

Good for Cholesterol

As said above, if you pay attention to the quality of the fats you consume, you will see an improvement in cholesterol: you will see your good cholesterol (HDL: High-Density Lipoprotein) increase, while your bad cholesterol (LDL: Low-Density Lipoprotein) will decrease.

You will also notice an improvement in triglyceride levels, as well as an improvement in blood pressure. Blood pressure problems are usually caused by being overweight, and the ketogenic diet is intended to cause weight loss and therefore reduce blood pressure problems.

Foods Allowed In Keto Diet

To make the most of your diet, there are prohibited foods and others that are allowed, but in limited quantities. Here are the foods allowed in the ketogenic diet:

Food allowed in unlimited quantities

Lean or fatty meats

No matter which meat you choose, it contains no carbohydrates so that you can have fun! Pay attention to the quality of your heart and the amount of fat. Alternate between fatty meats and lean meats!

Here are some examples of lean meats:

Beef: sirloin steak, roast beef, 5% minced steak, roast, flank steak, tenderloin, grisons meat, tripe, kidneys

Horse: roti, steak

Pork: tenderloin, bacon, kidneys

Veal: cutlet, shank, tenderloin, sweetbread, liver

Chicken and turkey: cutlet, skinless thigh, ham

Rabbit

Here are some examples of fatty meats:

Lamb: leg, ribs, brain

Beef: minced steak 10, 15, 20%, ribs, rib steak, tongue, marrow

Pork: ribs, brain, dry ham, black pudding, white pudding, bacon, terrine, rillettes, salami, sausage, sausages, and merguez

Veal: roast, paupiette, marrow, brain, tongue, dumplings

Chicken and turkey: thigh with skin

Guinea fowl

Capon

Turkey

Goose: foie gras

Lean or fatty fish

The fish does not contain carbohydrates so that you can consume unlimited! As with meat, there are lean fish and fatty fish, pay attention to the amount of fat you eat and remember to vary your intake of fish. Oily fish have the advantage of containing a lot of good cholesterol, so it is beneficial for protection against cardiovascular disease! It will be advisable to consume fatty fish more than lean fish to be able to manage your protein intake: if you consume bony fish, you will have a significant protein intake and little lipids, whereas, with fatty fish, you will have a balanced protein and fat intake!

Here are some examples of lean fish:

- Cod
- Colin
- Sea bream
- Whiting
- Sole
- Turbot
- Limor career
- Location
- Pike
- Ray

Here are some examples of oily fish:

- Swordfish

- Salmon

- Tuna

- Trout

- Monkfish

- Herring

- Mackerel

- Cod

- Sardine

Eggs

The eggs contain no carbohydrates, so you can consume as much as you want. It is often said that eggs are full of cholesterol and that you have to limit their intake, but the more cholesterol you eat, the less your body will produce by itself! Also, it's not just low-quality cholesterol, so that you can consume 6 per week without risk! And if you want to eat more but you are afraid of your cholesterol, and I have not convinced you, remove the yellow!

Vegetables and raw vegetables

Yes, you can eat vegetables... But you have to be careful which ones: you can eat leafy vegetables (salad, spinach, kale, red cabbage, Chinese cabbage...) and flower vegetables (cauliflower, broccoli, romanesco cabbage...) as well as avocado, cucumbers, zucchini or leeks, which do not contain many carbohydrates.

The oils

It's oil, so it's only fat, so it's unlimited to eat, but choose your oil wisely! Prefer olive oil, rapeseed, nuts, sunflower or sesame, for example!

Foods authorized in moderate quantities.

The cold cuts

As you know, there is bad cholesterol in cold meats, so you will need to moderate your intake: eat it occasionally!

Fresh cheeses and plain yogurts

Consume with moderation because they contain carbohydrates.

Nuts and oilseeds

They have low levels of carbohydrates but are rich in saturated fatty acids, that's why they should moderate their consumption. Choose almonds, hazelnuts, Brazil nuts or pecans.

Coconut (in oil, cream or milk)

It contains saturated fatty acids, that's why we limit its consumption. Cream and coconut oil have a lot of medium-chain triglycerides (MCTs), which increase the level of ketones, essential to stay in ketosis.

Berries and red fruits

They contain carbohydrates in reasonable quantities, but you should not abuse them to avoid ketosis (blueberries, blackberries, raspberries...).

Low-carb fruits

Some fruits contain few carbohydrates and can therefore be eaten occasionally, such as lemon or rhubarb.

CHAPTER 10:

Body Changes After 50, What Changes in the Women's Body?

As I have said earlier that you need to learn some things when you are starting with the ketogenic diet. For the most part, you need to know how to calculate your carbs and keep track of ketosis.

Calculating the carbs will let you make quick decisions and also plan. For instance, if there is an event that you need to attend down, the line says after a week. And you know that you won't get much choice of food that you can eat there, you can make sure that you have enough carbs already eaten beforehand. So that even if you do not eat anything or take a bite or two, the overall levels do not vary.

Although the best thing is to make sure that you are eating the right amount of nutrients, both micro and macro, every day, but in a situation like this, you can make appropriate arrangements provided you know how much diet you need to take.

More importantly, calories matter more on a keto diet. The USDA regulated that a woman of age between 50 to 60 needs up to 2200 calories every day. And the ones who are aged above 70 need 2000 calories per day. The cycle of calorie intake varies with age, height, weight, mass, and many other aspects.

In the later stages of life, this calorie intake is less because of the lower muscle mass, increased intensity of activity, and reduction basal metabolic rate. On the contrary, higher muscle mass means more calories are required to burn that extra fat.

In my opinion, every single woman should go for a keto diet when they cross the 50 years mark. This is because, after this age, you will need such a diet plan which accounts for each and everything that goes on inside the body. But, most importantly, it keeps the weight in check, takes care of the skin, and leads to a more active lifestyle. All of which are the central pillars of support in a ketogenic diet.

I have been asked several times that when the ketosis will begin or after how many months will my fat start burning. Well, there is no one response to this question. It depends and varies as per the individual.

Entering the stage of ketosis means that your body is not getting enough carbs or proteins to burn and that it is now using fats to get energy. To make this possible, the liver produces ketones that catalyze the fat burning process. Hence, when you need to know whether or not you have entered ketosis, track the level of ketones in the body. Keeping an eye on this level will help you get the right picture.

Other than this, weight loss, an increased tendency to drink more water, and cramps. I know getting muscle cramps is not a good thing. But when you are on a ketogenic diet, there is a vulnerability of imbalance in electrolyte levels of the body. Further, it can cause such spasms and cramps. Some of the crucial electrolytes are calcium, sodium, potassium, and magnesium. Whatever dish you choose to consume, make sure that you are getting enough of these electrolytes as to avoid getting into cramps and all.

The kind of diet that you were on before the keto diet also makes a difference in the time when you enter ketosis. For instance, if you have been eating a food that was rich in carbohydrates, it can take a bit longer than those who were consuming a lesser amount of carbs beforehand. This is because, in a ketogenic diet, the body does not rely upon carbs or sugars to get energy. Instead, they are now dependent on ketones, which will convert the fat into an energy source.

And one of the most significant adverse outcomes of this stress eating is obesity and other related issues. The woman that I support and start with this new lifestyle has also seen a lot in their lives that their mind is devoid of all such feelings, which can disrupt the practicing of the keto diet.

Other than this, you will also see various types of ingredients and food types that you can eat in a keto diet. There are multiple misnomers out there regarding this diet. I hope to clear them all in here.

CHAPTER 11:

Ketogenic Diet and Menopause

For aging women, menopause will bring severe changes and challenges, but a ketogenic diet can help you effortlessly switch gears to continue enjoying a healthy and happy life. Menopause can alter hormone levels in women, which in turn affects the brain's ability and cognitive abilities. Also, due to the lower production of estrogen and progesterone, your sex drive is lowered, and you suffer from sleep and mood problems. Let's take a look at how a ketogenic diet will help resolve these side effects.

1. Enhanced cognitive functions

Usually, the hormone estrogen ensures a constant flow of glucose to your brain. But after menopause, estrogen levels begin to drop dramatically, as does the amount of glucose in bran. As a result, the available power of your brain will start to deteriorate. However, by following the ketogenic diet for women over 50, the problem of glucose intake is avoided. This results in improved cognitive functions and brain activity.

2. Hormonal balance

Usually, women experience significant menopausal symptoms due to hormonal imbalances. The ketogenic diet for women over 50 works by stabilizing these imbalances like estrogen. This helps show tolerable minor menopausal symptoms, such as hot flashes. The keto diet also balances insulin and blood sugar levels and helps control insulin sensitivity.

3. Intense sex drive

The ketogenic diet increases the absorption of vitamin D, which is essential for improving sexual desire. Vitamin D ensures stable levels of testosterone and other sex hormones that could become unstable due to low testosterone levels.

4. Better sleep

Glucose alters your blood sugar levels, which in turn leads to a low quality of sleep. Along with other symptoms of menopause, sleeping well becomes a big problem as you age. The ketogenic diet for women over 50 not only balances blood glucose levels, but also stabilizes other hormones such as cortisol, melatonin, and serotonin that ensure better and better sleep.

5. Reduces inflammation

Menopause can increase inflammation levels by leaving potentially harmful invaders in our system, resulting in unpleasant and painful symptoms. The ketogenic diet for women over 50 uses healthy anti-inflammatory fats to reduce inflammation and pain in the joints and bones.

6. Fill your brain

Did you know that your brain is made up of 60% fat or more? This means that more fat is needed to maintain optimal function. In other words, the ketones in the ketogenic diet serve as an energy source that fuels brain cells.

7. Nutrient deficiencies

Aging women tend to have more significant deficiencies in essential nutrients such as iron deficiency, leading to mental confusion and fatigue. Vitamin B12 deficiency, leading to neurological conditions such as dementia. Fat lack, which can cause problems with knowledge, skin, vision, and vitamin D deficiency that not only causes cognitive decline in older adults and increases the risk of heart disease but also contributes to the risk of developing cancer. On a ketogenic diet, high-quality protein provides excellent and adequate sources of these essential nutrients.

CHAPTER 12:

How to Get Started with Keto Diet After 50

Approach to be adopted

Here are a few proposals that may assist you with arriving at your objectives on a keto diet:

To start with, ensure that you're following something beyond your carbs. Keto is minimal in carb (20 g or less every day as you're as of now doing), yet it has moderate protein (50–75 grams for every day for ladies), and high fat (in any event a 1:1 up to a 1:2 proportion of protein to fat). In case you're not previously following your protein and fat alongside your carbs, start.

The protein and fat are particularly significant in case you're attempting to get "tore" as you state. You need the protein to construct muscle and the fat to give you vitality to work out.

Keep in mind, on keto, you're changing your body from consuming carbs and sugars for fuel to using body fats for energy - which is better for your body, your cerebrum, and for work out - however, in case you're not giving enough fats for your body, you won't have sufficient energy to consume.

Furthermore, since you express that you've generally been thin, you likely don't have a lot, assuming any, and abundance fat on your body to consume, so you certainly need to get the fat in your nourishment consistently.

Second, you state that you're on a considerable shortfall. You most likely don't have to follow your calories at all in case you're eating keto effectively. Keto depends on tuning in to your body - eating when you're eager and halting eating when you're full.

This sounds basic; however, it conflicts with what most of us have learned and done for our entire lives - eating three suppers every day at recommended times and cleaning our plates whether we're ravenous. What's more, since you'll be eating significantly more fat than you're utilized to and not a lot of carbs by any stretch of the imagination (which causes desires and sugar crashes), you'll feel full quicker. For more, so you won't eat to such an extent, and you won't have any desire to eat as frequently, which implies the calories will deal with themselves. (Numerous individuals on the keto diet just eat a couple of suppers daily since they simply aren't ravenous more than that.)

For you explicitly, since you're attempting to pick up muscle and you're as of now thin, you unquestionably don't should be on a calorie-confined or calorie shortage diet - and you may need to eat close to the top finish of the protein to fat proportion to ensure your body has the vitality it needs. So, eat that great fat and protein and appreciate them!

Third, one of the general most significant advantages of keto is getting your body into ketosis - which is the consequence of changing your body from consuming carbs and sugars to consuming fats. For competitors, this is fundamental with the goal that you can have the most elevated conceivable execution. When your body is in ketosis, you'll notice numerous advantages that will assist you with your exhibition - more vitality, better rest, more stamina, and so forth. So, it's incredibly significant that you see all the segments of the keto method for eating with the goal that you can get your body into ketosis.

For more insights regarding eating keto, look at this asset, CRACK the Keto CODE, which contains bunches of extraordinary information including what nourishments are ideal for wearing on keto and what food sources are perfect for maintaining a strategic distance from, how to track (and change) your macros, what are electrolytes and for what reason are they so significant (particularly as a competitor this will be a serious deal for you), and even some incredible keto plans.

Fasting yes or no?

The topic of fasting is controversial. Indeed, fasting is good if it is done the correct way. Unreasonable fasting isn't acceptable.

An average individual ordinarily eats three suppers every day and snacks in the middle. The gastric discharging time after a healthy feast is 4 hours. Yet, before the nourishment is exhausted out, we nibble/eat more. We are continually keeping our digestive organs grinding away. Fasting allows our digestion tracts to rest. Also, there are many poisons created in our body, and they never persuade an opportunity to be purged.

Thirdly, it fortifies your body and improves resistance, for, during this period, you have washed down yourself, yet have ingested just simple squeezes that get retained no problem at all. You retain everything. Also, afterward, you feel spotless, sound, crisp and revived. It sure is a great idea to watch a quick to detoxify yourself on more than one occasion per year.

Before I talk about something which accomplishes work – would we be able to pause for a minute to consider this insane weight control plans us catch wind of? It appears each week the web has some new prevailing fashion diet, detox or quick. If even 10% of the guarantees they make are genuine, we'd never need another again. Everybody swears their eating routine is the one which works. Everyone has their little snare.

People fast to get in shape. Others do fast to detox their bodies, or for strict reasons. In case you're fasting to get in shape, you might need to reevaluate. The weight reduction may not last after you complete the process of fasting. On the off chance that you will likely detox your body, you should realize that your body detoxes itself typically.

Why Can Fasting for Weight Loss Backfire?

At the point when you eat short of what you need, and you get more fit, your body goes into a starvation mode. To spare vitality, your digestion eases back down. At the point when you're finished fasting, and you return to your standard eating regimen, you may recover the weight you lost, to say the very least.

On a fast, your body alters by checking your craving so that you will feel less eager from the start. Be that as it may, when you have quit fasting, you're craving fires up back. You may feel hungrier and be bound to indulge.

Fasting each other day has comparative outcomes. It assists individuals with shedding pounds, yet not for long. Be that as it may, the weight reduction didn't last after some time.

Is Fasting Safe?

Fasting for a couple of days likely won't hurt a great many people who are reliable, if they don't get dried out. Yet, fasting for extended periods is awful for you.

Your body needs nutrients, minerals, and different supplements from nourishment to remain sound. On the off chance that you don't get enough, you can have manifestations, for example, weakness, wooziness, blockage, drying out, and not having the option to endure cold temperatures. Fasting too long can be perilous. Try not to fast, in any event, for a brief timeframe, on the off chance that you have diabetes since it can prompt risky dunks and spikes in glucose. Others who shouldn't fast are ladies who are pregnant or breastfeeding, anybody with an incessant sickness, the old, and kids.

Before you go on another eating regimen, especially one that includes fasting, inquire as to whether it's a decent decision for you. You can likewise approach your primary care physician for a referral to an enrolled dietitian, who can tell you the best way to structure a smart dieting plan.

CHAPTER 13:

The Keto Diet Mindset

Like any other life-transforming endeavor, the keto diet regimen is dependent on your mindset. You must be prepared to face the emotional, physical, and psychological obstacles that will arise in the course of achieving your goals. This underpins the impact the diet will have on your life. In this regard, one of the fundamental elements of keto is a mindset that is equipped to deal with many obstacles and challenges.

For some, the desire to lose weight is the underlying impetus, while others are motivated by the goal of living healthier lives. In some cases, a person may be forced to consider a diet change for medical or biological reasons. Regardless of the motivation, maintaining the right mindset always determines the success of a change in diet. In this regard, attaining an appropriate attitude is the first step towards initiating and benefitting from a keto-based diet.

The Right Mindset for a Keto Diet

When beginning a keto diet, the first phase of your journey must be adopting an appropriate mindset that will allow you to make this lifestyle change successfully. While you might set your goals right from the start, you must consider that your energy and enthusiasm is likely to wane over time. For most people, this results in failure, which is then translated into frustration and the loss of confidence in the ketogenic diet. By emotionally and psychologically preparing oneself for the journey ahead, it is possible to achieve this feat quite easily.

You must first acknowledge and accept in your mind that the diet does work and that you can experience its impact on your life. This is the first and most crucial thought process that will help you actively and judiciously stick to the plan. If you have tried other diet plans in the past with little success, this particular thought process may be hard to come by. However, by shifting your focus to scientific and factual material regarding the diet, you may begin to appreciate its efficacy.

The capacity to individually internalize this concept forms the basis of the essential mindset for a keto diet. By eliminating any form of doubt in your mind concerning the benefits and impact of a keto diet, you set yourself up for success. This is because it helps you stay focused on the outcome while ignoring the day to day challenges and distractions that will undoubtedly arise. Internalization and appreciation of the benefits and effectiveness of the keto diet create the necessary momentum needed to consistently adhere to the stipulations that come with the implementation of the diet.

The elimination of excuses is also fundamental if you are to realize the benefits of a keto diet. For most people, dietary changes are seen as significant transformations that occur overnight. For a woman in her 50s, this can prove daunting and even scary. When you have already lived on a different diet for half a century, you have an internal block that causes you to doubt your ability to change the content of your diet. You are likely to come up with numerous excuses and justifications as to why such a diet may not work for you. If you are looking at a keto diet as a total overhaul of how you are a person, then there is a higher likelihood you will find the endeavor too arduous even to try.

By holding onto the notion, a keto diet is only successful when drastic and dramatic changes are made in your life, you save yourself back with your thoughts. In most cases, this line of thinking should raise the red flag of fear and unnecessary excuses. While your former attempts at dieting may have informed such notions, you must approach a keto diet with a fresh and curious mind.

It is also essential to approach the keto diet as a new partner that will bring you much-awaited love, compassion, and care. In this case, therefore, you must assume a sense of self-love and care to ensure that it works. Day-to-day interactions and experiences can often impose a sense of negativity and self-loathing. In failing to accomplish various goals, meet specific demands, or achieve individual personal, professional, or social goals, the burden of guilt and self-hate is likely to emerge.

Such a state of mind is limited in numerous ways, and as such, it cannot achieve the desired frequency of caring for itself. Once you learn to be kind and patient with yourself, you realize life has its ups and downs. Regardless of these challenges, you must give yourself the time and space to fail, learn, and grow as you go. The self-care mindset is crucial for effectiveness on the keto diet. By appreciating and loving yourself, you initiate a process in which your well-being is paramount to your survival. As such, you are ready to undertake any efforts whatsoever to improve the quality of your life. A sense of purpose and limitlessness becomes a constant aspect of your life, and as such, you can see your goals and ambitions through.

As is the case, with most new things, encounters, and experiences, you are likely to feel the need to remind yourself of the feeling continuously. For instance, when you buy a new phone, you may not want to put it down even as you explore its features and quirks. Over time your adoration for the new item may turn into an obsession or compulsive behavior that can be hard to break. The same analogy works when it comes to dieting. In setting out to try a new diet, as is the case with a keto diet, you may fixate on the expected outcomes and results. It is essential to note the fact that while your weight may be slow to change, there is a likelihood your muscle structure will have a change in terms of getting leaner. By moving away from the metric-tracking mentality, you allow yourself the time to acclimate to the diet and notice the overall changes it brings about in your physical, psychological, and emotional well-being rather than fixating on the pounds lost or gained.

Cognitively preparing for the long-haul is also vital in achieving the goals and benefits of a keto diet.

The best way to appreciate a ketogenic diet is by looking at it as a lifestyle change rather than a change in dietary intakes. While the benefits of the diet are factual and well documented, they take time to come about. Most people, however, hold the belief that a keto diet is a quick fix solution that allows them to transform their health, weight, and body shape within weeks or months. Having gleaned information from various media platforms, such individuals are quick to adopt the diet with the hope of having an overnight transformation.

The quick-fix mindset is one of the surest ways of failing in your pursuit to experience the benefits of a ketogenic diet. You must be willing to endure for the long-term goals while celebrating the short-term gains. A two-week on a two-month keto diet may accord you the much need weight loss. However, such changes are likely to disappear just as fast in the absence of long-term commitment.

Strategies to Develop the Right Mindset for a Keto Diet

Having understood the dynamics surrounding the perfect keto diet mindset, you may wonder how you will achieve such a feat. In other words, you want to establish the actual and practical steps towards developing a paradigm shift. The fields of psychology and behavioral science have been instrumental in expanding knowledge and information surrounding human behavior.

- Being aware of your Inner and Outer Surrounding

In this regard, the first and most important strategy is raising one's awareness of both inner and outer surroundings. With food as a crucial trigger of behavior and habit, maintaining a sense of awareness regarding your thought patterns, cravings, and moment to moment, activities offer the first step towards mastering your dietary behavior.

In an effort to build upon your awareness, you might need to keep a journal as one way of keeping track of your thought patterns and activities. With this in place, it becomes easier to review your day while noticing recurrent thoughts and activities. This will prove crucial in helping you plan your day with respect to meals and exercises while keeping track of your dietary intake. Most importantly, however, is the fact it will help you in cultivating the discipline needed with respect to keeping track of your consumption patterns.

- Keeping an Open Mind

With your awareness in check, you will need to strive to have an open mind considering the diverse results of the keto diet form one person to another. In an effort to establish a keto-diet mindset, it will be imperative that you remain as open as possible to new ideas, experiments, lessons, disappointments, and victories. Having a fixed mindset regarding the outcomes and expectations from a keto diet serves no purpose at all. You should not approach a keto diet experience with pre-established ideas and notions.

- The Willingness to put in the Work

While most media depictions of keto diets revolve around quick and short-term gains associated with the change, the reality is far more arduous and long. Beyond the glamour of abs, swift loss of weight, and bright and glowing skin, you must be willing to invest your time and resources to realize your health and diet goals. This translates to creating time to educate yourself and gain the knowledge and skills necessary to actualize your keto diet dream.

- The readiness to make Changes in Your Life

The attainment of a keto diet mindset is also contingent upon your ability to make changes across various areas of your life. Having appreciated the food and eating as habitual behaviors, you must be will to overcome and transform various aspects of your life if you are to enjoy the benefits of a keto diet. This requires a comprehensive audit of your life with a focus on your habits and behavior over time. Your ability to change primarily lies in your comprehension of the factors around your day-to-day life.

As your work towards achieving your healthy diet goal, the need for change will arise from every other corner. Any form of resistance from any faculty of your life may result in unprecedented outcomes with respect to your dieting. In essence, in committing to a keto diet, you must be ready to endure various uncomfortable experiences in the short-term.

- Visualization

Visualization entails creating mental images of yourself in a healthier, leaner, and more confident state. This means taking time to capture all the upsides that will result from your efforts to transform yourself. You will need to look at the type of relationships you will have, the health benefits associated with the changes you make, and, most importantly, what it will take for you to achieve your goals.

CHAPTER 14:

Common Mistakes to Avoid

Do you feel like you are giving your all to the Keto diet, but you still aren't seeing the results you want? You are measuring ketones, working out, and counting your macros, but you still aren't losing the weight you want. Here are the most common mistakes that most people make when beginning the Keto diet.

1. Too Many Snacks

There are many snacks you can enjoy while following the Keto diet, like nuts, avocado, seeds, and cheese. But, snacking can be an easy way to get too many calories into the diet while giving your body an easy fuel source besides stored fat. Snacks need to be only used if you frequently hunger between meals. If you aren't extremely hungry, let your body turn to your stored fat for its fuel between meals instead of dietary fat.

2. Not Consuming Enough Fat

The ketogenic diet isn't all about low carbs. It's also about high fats. You need to be getting about 75 percent of your calories from healthy fats, five percent from carbs, and 20 percent from protein. Fat makes you feel fuller longer, so if you eat the correct amount, you will minimize your carb cravings, and this will help you stay in ketosis. This will help your body burn fat faster.

3. Consuming Excessive Calories

You may hear people say you can eat what you want on the Keto diet as long as it is high in fat. Even though we want that to be true, it is very misleading. Healthy fats need to make up the biggest part of your diet. If you eat more calories than what you are burning, you will gain weight, no matter what you eat, because these excess calories get stored as fat. An average adult only needs about 2,000 calories each day, but this will vary based on many factors like activity level, height, and gender.

4. Consuming a lot of Dairies

For many people, dairy can cause inflammation and keeps them from losing weight. Dairy is a combo food meaning it has carbs, protein, and fats. If you eat a lot of cheese as a snack for the fat content, you are also getting a dose of carbs and protein with that fat. Many people can tolerate dairy, but moderation is the key.

5. Consuming a lot of Protein

The biggest mistake that most people make when just beginning the Keto diet is consuming too much protein. Excess protein gets converted into glucose in the body called gluconeogenesis. When following a ketogenic diet, gluconeogenesis happens at different rates to keep the body function. Our bodies don't need a lot of carbs, but we do need glucose. You can eat absolute zero carbs, and through gluconeogenesis, your body will convert other substances into glucose to be used as fuel. This is why carbs only make up five percent of your macros. Some parts of our bodies need carbs to survive, like the kidney, medulla, and red blood cells. With gluconeogenesis, our bodies make and stores extra glucose as glycogen just in case supplies become too low.

In a normal diet, when carbs are always available, gluconeogenesis happens slowly because the need for glucose is extremely low. Our body runs on glucose and will store excess protein and carbs as fat.

6. Not Getting Enough Water

Water is crucial for your body. Water is needed for all your body does, and this includes burning fat. If you don't drink enough water, it can cause your metabolism to slow down, and this can halt your weight loss. Drinking 64 ounces or one-half gallon every day will help your body burn fat, flush out toxins, and circulate nutrients.

7. Consuming Too Many Sweets

Some people might indulge in Keto brownies and Keto cookies that are full of sugar substitutes just because their net carb content is low, but you have to remember that you are still eating calories. Eating sweets might increase your carb cravings. Keto sweets are great on occasion; they don't need to be a staple in the diet.

8. Not Getting Enough Sleep

Getting plenty of sleep is needed in order to lose weight effectively. Without the right amount of sleep, your body will feel stressed, and this could result in your metabolism slowing down. It might cause it to store fat instead of burning fat. When you feel tired, you are more tempted to drink more lattes for energy, eat a snack to give you an extra boost, or order takeout rather than cooking a healthy meal.

9. Low on Electrolytes

Most people will experience the Keto flu when you begin this diet. This happens for two reasons when your body changes from burning carbs to burning fat, your brain might not have enough energy, and this, in turn, can cause grogginess, headaches, and nausea. You could be dehydrated, and your electrolytes might be low since the Keto diet causes you to urinate often.

Getting the Keto flu is a great sign that you are heading in the right direction. You can lessen these symptoms by drinking more water or taking supplements that will balance your electrolytes.

10. Consuming Hidden Carbs

Many foods look like they are low carb, but they aren't. You can find carbs in salad dressings, sauces, and condiments. Be sure to check nutrition labels before you try new foods to make sure it doesn't have any hidden sugar or carbs. It just takes a few seconds to skim the label, and it might be the difference between whether or not you'll lose weight.

If you have successfully ruled out all of the above, but you still aren't losing weight, you might need to talk with your doctor to make sure you don't have any health problems that could be preventing your weight loss. This can be frustrating, but stick with it, stay positive, and stay in the game. When the Keto diet is done correctly, it is one of the best ways to lose weight.

CHAPTER 15:

28-day Meal Plan

For people who are new to the Keto Diet, the way to meal plan might seem both full of possibilities and full of pitfalls. The reality is that the best solution is the KISS method (Keep It Simple Stupid). The key to this diet is to make sure that you are keeping everything within your proper ratios. This is a really important part of the Keto Diet when you stay in the ratios that you need to be in, what will happen is that you can make sure that you get the most out of your diet.

However, this is just the first step, the next thing to think about is what exactly you can eat? Well, there is good news, there are tons of options with proteins. This is a way that you can make life easy on yourself. One of the sources of protein should be eggs. They are really easy and versatile, and eggs are also ridiculously cheap. Another great idea is using seafood. The smaller types of seafood are better; for example, sardines are a great source of protein because they are high in Omega-3, which has a ton of benefits for the body. Some other seafood includes salmon, shrimp, cod, and even oysters. That said, many of these different meats can get expensive. Also, if you are able to get grass-fed or organic meat, that is always better than going with the conventional types, which means that you have a greater amount of fat content.

Here are some sources of protein – again, adjust if you are on a budget:

- Grass-fed beef
- Seafood that is wild-caught
- Pork; preferably pasture-raised
- Eggs – vegetarian diet is the standard
- Grass-fed chicken
- Yogurt in moderation

Oils also have some very interesting properties as well, and what you are cooking with will definitely affect your progress on the Keto Diet. One of the great tips for adding flavor is to cook your greens in Extra Virgin Olive Oil or bacon fat. This is a great way to get a flavor. Avocado oil and olive oil also work well with salad dressings. When you decide that you want to marinate food, be sure to use avocado oil. Butter, of course, is wonderful to cook with and uncured bacon is both a great thing to render fat from and also to eat. Also, the rendered fat has a higher smoke point, so you can feel assured that you won't have to deal with the oxidized LDL cholesterol that is responsible for the hardening of arteries, the building of plaque, and this is what causes heart disease as well.

Choosing your vegetables is also very important, and the thing that you want to do is get dark leafy greens like spinach and kale. There are others as well, such as bok choy. The good news is when you are using butter and bacon fat for cooking these vegetables, you will enjoy their flavors. These vegetables are loaded with different nutrients that your body needs, including calcium and other vitamins and minerals that will make up for any deficiencies that you may have had. Plus, they have amazingly complex flavors and can be used in so many different ways.

There are plenty of other vegetables to use as well, so don't get caught in a kale and spinach cycle because that results in the building up of different oxalates, and the end results are kidney stones. No one wants to deal with that. Mushrooms are also good and have a low amount of net carbs; asparagus, Brussel sprouts, zucchini, onions, and bell peppers all do the job too. Throw in some balsamic vinegar, and you have some excellent flavors. These veggies also tolerate the grill really well too.

The fruit is something that should be used in moderation, and the key with fruit is making sure that you are all about the berries. Blackberries, raspberries, blueberries and strawberries are ideal because they are both high in fiber and also in antioxidants. Furthermore, win and dark chocolate also have great power with the Keto Diet as well. There are lots of other things to consider too. Make sure that the fruit is lower in sugar because this will avoid the increase in the insulin, and that creates problems with the Keto Diet.

Once you have the food that you want to eat, the next step is making sure that you are cooking it the way that you want. There are some different methods that you should use. The first is that you want to make sure that you are going one of three ways. The best methods are using a pressure cooker, the stovetop, or firing up the grill.

There are lots of interesting ideas as well. Bone broth is something that is really fun to make during meal prep, and it is done with the pressure cooker. There are also dishes like Keto lasagna, pulled pork, keto cheesecake, ground beef dishes, hard-boiled eggs and even veggie lasagna. When you reflect on where you were and how far you have come, you will notice that you were eating a bunch of starches, including pasta, rice, mac and cheese, baked potatoes, etc. The pressure cooker is one of the best ways that you can prepare food in a healthy way, and it makes life so much easier.

Here is a 28-day meal plan for weight loss and boost energy for breakfast, lunch, dinner, and snacks.

Days	Breakfast	Lunch	Dinner	Dessert
1	Bacon Cheese Waffles	Mediterranean Keto Dish	Beef-Stuffed Mushroom	Quick Rhum Cocoa Truffles
2	Keto Breakfast Cheesecake	Spicy Zoodles with Cheese	Rib Roast	Raspberry Cheesecake
3	Egg-Crust Pizza	Spicy Ground Turkey Dish	Buffalo Chicken Soup	Chocolate Cake
4	Breakfast Roll-Ups	Hungarian Pork Stew	Sweet &Sour Pork	Coconut Cocoa Brownies
5	Basic Opie Rolls	Easy Zucchini Noodles	Grilled Pork with Salsa	Orange Lime Pudding
6	Cream Cheese Pancake	Keto Cheese Potato	Weekend Dinner Stew	Almond Cocoa Spread
7	Blueberry Coconut Porridge	Keto Veggie Dish	Chicken Pesto	Chia Vanilla Custard
8	Cauliflower Hash Browns	Delicious Keto Potato Wedges	Garlic Parmesan Chicken Wings	Walnut Pumpkin Mug Cake

9	Keto Rolls	Easy Jalapeno Rings	Crispy Baked Shrimp	Chocolate Cake with Vanilla Glaze
10	Almond Flour Pancakes	Hot Spicy Chicken	Herbed Mediterranean Fish Fillet	Rum Truffles
11	Avocado Toast	Broccoli and Turkey Dish	Mushroom Stuffed with Ricotta	Mint Cake
12	Chicken Avocado Egg Bacon Salad	Easy Mayo Salmon	Thai Chopped Salad	Vanilla Cherry Panna Cotta
13	Bacon-Wrapped Chicken Breast	Delicious Tomato Basil Soup	Lemon & Rosemary Salmon	Mocha Pots de Creme
14	Egg Salad	Keto Teriyaki Chicken	Ideal Cold Weather Stew	Lemon Cake with Berry Syrup
15	Blueberry Muffins	Lime Chicken with Coleslaw	Baked Lemon & Pepper Chicken	Easy Rhum Cheesecake
16	Bacon Hash	Beef Satay and Peanut Sauce	Skillet Chicken either White Wine Sauce	Chocolate Cake
17	Bagels with Cheese	Mini Meatloaves	Stir Fry Kimchi and Pork Belly	Chia Vanilla Custard
18	Cauli Flitters	Greek Meatballs Salad	Lemon Butter Sauce with Fish	Rum Truffles
19	Scrambled Eggs	Low Carb Chicken Philly Cheesesteak	Slow Cooker Taco Soup	Mint Cake
20	Frittata with Spinach	Curry Soup	Bacon Bleu Cheese Filled Eggs	Walnut Pumpkin Mug Cake
21	Cheese Omelet	Chicken Nuggets	Mexican Pork Stew	Raspberry Cheesecake
22	Capicola Egg Cups	Winter Comfort Stew	Chicken with Lemon and Garlic	Orange Lime Pudding
23	Basic Opie Rolls	Chicken Kurma	Chicken Pot Pie in a Slow Cooker	Lemon Cake with Berry Syrup
24	Cream Cheese Pancake	Garlic Pork Loin	Cheese Cauli Breadsticks	Chocolate Cake with Vanilla Glaze
25	Keto Rolls	Spinach Stuffed Chicken Breasts	Yummy Eggplant with Cheese	Vanilla Cherry Panna Cotta

26	Avocado Toasts	Keto Reuben Skillet	Yellow Chicken Stew	Mocha Pots de Creme
27	Egg Salad	Chicken Enchilada Soup	Zesty Avocado and Lettuce Salad	Easy Rum Cheesecake
28	Bacon Hash	Beef Stir Fry	Wedding Soup	Coconut Cocoa Brownies

CHAPTER 16:

Keto Diet Shopping List for Women Over 50

Week 1

Poultry, Meat, & Seafood

4 (1½-pound) Cornish game hens

1 (4-pound) grass-fed whole chicken

3 pounds grass-fed chicken breast

11 (6-ounces) grass-fed boneless skinless chicken breasts

3 pounds grass-fed boneless, skinless chicken breasts

4 (6-ounce) grass-fed boneless, skinless chicken breast halves

8 (6-ounce) grass-fed skinless chicken thighs

1 (9-pound) whole turkey

1 (7-pound) bone-in turkey breast

3 pounds lean ground turkey

2½ pounds grass-fed beef chuck roast

1 (3-pound) grass-fed center-cut beef tenderloin roast

Vegetables

Six heads broccoli

2 (12-ounce) packages riced cauliflower

One pumpkin

Ten zucchinis

2 (10-ounce) packages frozen spinach

1 (16-ounce) bag frozen chopped spinach

Ten bags fresh spinach

One bag fresh arugula

Two bags fresh baby spinach

VICTORIA WILLS

8 green bell pepper

5 red bell pepper

1 carrot

Fruit

2 avocados

1 bag fresh strawberries

1 bag frozen strawberries

4 bags fresh raspberries

1 bag fresh cranberries

Dairy Products

12 tubs butter

1 tub unsalted butter

6 tubs plain Greek yogurt

4 jars mayonnaise

1 tub sour cream

11 tubs heavy cream

4 tubs heavy whipping cream

8 packages cream cheese

7 packages Parmesan cheese

Seasonings & Spices

2 bottles salt

2 bottles ground black pepper

1 bottle pumpkin pie spice

1 bottle ground allspice

1 bottle ground cinnamon

1 bottle ground nutmeg

1 bottle ground cloves

1 bottle ground cardamom

1 bottle ground ginger

1 bottle cumin seeds

1 bottle coriander seeds

1 bottle mustard seed

Extras

97 organic eggs

9 cans unsweetened almond milk

7 cans unsweetened coconut milk

1 jar Italian dressing

2 bottles of olive oil

1 bottle of coconut oil

1 bottle sesame oil

1 bottle MCT oil

1 bag almond flour

1 bag superfine blanched almond flour

1 bag coconut flour

1 bag arrowroot starch

Week 2

Poultry, Meat, & Seafood

1 (10-pound) grass-fed prime rib roast

2 (4-ounce) grass-fed beef tenderloin steaks

4 (6-ounces) grass-fed beef tenderloin filets

2 ½ pounds grass-fed ground beef

1 (5-pound) grass-fed bone-in leg of lamb, trimmed

2 (2½-pounds) grass-fed racks of lamb

1 pound grass-fed ground lamb

1 pound pork loin

1 pound pork tenderloin

4 pounds pork rib

Vegetables

3 pounds asparagus

1 bag fresh white mushrooms

3 bags fresh button mushrooms

½ cup Kalamata olives

6 bags tomatoes

1 bag cherry tomatoes

5 large English cucumbers

12 yellow onions

11 celery stalks

5 heads garlic

Fruit

2 avocados

1 bag fresh strawberries

1 bag frozen strawberries

4 bags fresh raspberries

1 bag fresh cranberries

Dairy Products

1 package Parmigiano Reggiano cheese

7 packages cheddar cheese

1 package sharp cheddar cheese

7 packages mozzarella cheese

2 packages Swiss cheese

1 package provolone cheese

2 packages ricotta cheese

1 package feta cheese

1 package cottage cheese

Seasonings & Spices

1 bottle anise seeds

1 bottle whole allspice berries

1 bottle fenugreek seeds

1 bottle ground cumin

1 bottle ground coriander

1 bottle dehydrated onion flakes

1 bottle granulated garlic

1 bottle garlic powder

1 bottle onion powder

1 bottle ground turmeric

1 bottle curry powder

1 bottle garam masala

Extras

1 bag xanthan gum

1 bottle organic baking powder

1 bottle baking soda

1 bag flaxseed meal

1 bag chia seeds

1 bag poppy seeds

1 bag almonds

1 bag raw almonds1 bag pine nuts

1 bag walnuts

1 bag 70% dark chocolate chips

1 bag unsweetened vanilla whey protein powder

1 bottle matcha green tea powder

1 bottle cacao powder

1 bottle instant espresso powder

Week 3

Poultry, Meat, & Seafood

4 pounds lean ground pork

16 bacon slices

1 jar liver pate

6 (6-ounce) skinless, boneless salmon fillets

1 pound smoked salmon

1½ pounds skinless grouper fillets

1 (15-ounce) can water-packed tuna

Vegetables

15 lemons

5 limes

12 heads lettuce

1 fresh red chili

1 green chil

3 Serrano peppers

2 jalapeño peppers

7 bunches fresh parsley

6 bunches fresh dill

Fruit

2 avocados

1 bag fresh strawberries

1 bag frozen strawberries

4 bags fresh raspberries

1 bag fresh cranberries

Dairy Products

1 package Parmigiano Reggiano cheese

7 packages cheddar cheese

1 package sharp cheddar cheese

7 packages mozzarella cheese

2 packages Swiss cheese

1 package provolone cheese

2 packages ricotta cheese

1 package feta cheese

1 package cottage cheese

Seasonings & Spices

1 bottle paprika

1 bottle smoked paprika

1 bottle cayenne pepper

1 bottle red chili powder

1 bottle red pepper flakes

1 bottle chili flakes

1 bottle fennel seeds

1 bottle lemon pepper

1 bottle Italian seasoning

1 pack ranch seasoning mix

Extras

1 bottle instant coffee

1 tub almond butter

1 jar tahini

1 jar Dijon mustard

1 jar mustard powder

1 bottle chili sauce

1 bottle low-sodium soy sauce

1 bottle red boat fish sauce

1 bottle Worcestershire sauce

1 bottle liquid smoke

1 bottle organic vanilla extract

1 bottle organic lemon extract

2 bottles granulated erythritol

Week 4

Poultry, Meat, & Seafood

16 ounces canned tuna in olive oil

2 (1½-pound) wild-caught trout

5 pounds shrimp

1¼ pounds fresh scallops

¼ pound bay scallops

¼ pound fresh squid

¼ pound mussels

Vegetables

3 bunches fresh mint

1 bunch fresh chives

8 bunches fresh cilantro

20 bunches fresh basil

4 bunches fresh rosemary

2 bunches fresh thyme

2 bunches fresh oregano

2 bunches scallion

Fruit

2 avocados

1 bag fresh strawberries

1 bag frozen strawberries

4 bags fresh raspberries

1 bag fresh cranberries

Dairy Products

12 tubs butter

1 tub unsalted butter

6 tubs plain Greek yogurt

4 jars mayonnaise

1 tub sour cream

11 tubs heavy cream

4 tubs heavy whipping cream

8 packages cream cheese

7 packages Parmesan cheese

Seasonings & Spices

1 bottle poultry seasoning

1 bottle taco seasoning

1 bottle lemon-pepper seasoning

1 bottle dried parsley

1 bottle dried rosemary

1 bottle dried thyme

1 bottle dried basil1 bottle dried oregano

1 bottle dried sage

1 bottle dried marjoram

Extras

2 bottles powdered erythritol

1 bottle liquid stevia

1 bottle powdered stevia

1 bottle Yukon syrup

1 bottle organic apple cider vinegar

1 bottle balsamic vinegar

5 cans sugar-free tomato paste

1 jar sugar-free BBQ sauce

1 jar sugar-free ketchup

1 jar sugar-free HP steak sauce

1 can chopped green chilies

1 vanilla bean

CHAPTER 17:

Top 10 Healthy Foods You Must Eat and Enjoy as A Successful Ketogenic Dieter

Staying in ketosis by eating the right foods is key to healthy weight loss. It is important that you consume more healthy fats than protein to stay in this particular metabolic pathway. I will constantly stress the importance of following the percentage of 5% carbs, 20% protein, and 75% fats. This means that you need to build your meals around low carb vegetables, healthy oils, and moderate protein. Below are the foods that you can consume to drive ketosis.

• **Good fats:** Remember that not all fats are created equally. While some fats are bad, some are very healthy for the body. You need to consume more good fats in the ketogenic diet. Your options include MCT oil, coconut oil, butter, olive oil, ghee, avocado oil, and other dairy sources like unprocessed cheese and cream. Another good source of healthy fat is avocado.

• **Meat:** Choose from a selection of red meats, pork, chicken, turkey, and organ meats. Consume only a matchbox-sized portion for this diet regimen.

• **Fatty fish:** Fatty fish is a great source of fatty acids like Omega-3s that are precursors to ketones. Source them from trout, sardines, salmon, herring, and mostly cold-water fishes as they have more Omega-3s than other fishes.

• **Eggs:** Eggs are good sources of healthy fats and proteins.

• **Nuts and seeds:** Nuts and seeds are stapled food items among keto dieters. Have a steady supply of brazil nuts, almond nuts, walnuts, pumpkin seeds, chia seeds, and cashew nuts.

• **Vegetables growing above ground:** Low carb vegetables in the form of leafy greens, cucumbers, onions, tomatoes, broccoli, cauliflower, and peppers are allowed in this diet. Basically, all vegetables growing above ground (except some squash varieties and tomatoes) are mostly made up of fiber, water, and less sugar.

• **Berries:** While most fruits are high discouraged while following the ketogenic diet, there are low sugar fruits that you are allowed to eat, and these include blueberries, limes, lemons, apples, and strawberries.

• **Sweeteners:** Sweeteners sourced from sugar with a high glycemic index is bad for the ketogenic diet. However, allowed sweeteners include stevia, monk fruits, and erythritol.

• **Water:** Water is the most acceptable beverage in the ketogenic diet because it contains no calories. But if you are not such a big fan of this particular diet, you can always opt for other beverages such as tea, coffee, and red wine (occasionally).

• **Bone broth:** Bone broth is not only hydrating, but it is also chockfull of electrolytes, healthy fats, and nutrients. It is a great beverage to sip on the keto diet. For added fat, add a small dollop of butter to jump start ketosis.

Top 10 Foods You Definitely Must Avoid During Your Ketogenic Journey

The ketogenic diet is not rocket science. While it limits what type of foods that you can consume, it is not really difficult to eliminate certain food groups from your meals. Below are the types of foods that you need to avoid because they don't drive ketosis in the body.

- **Sugar of all types:** These include honey, maple syrup, white sugar, brown sugar, molasses, and fruit sugars.

- **Soda and fruit juice:** Soda and fruit juice (yes, even the natural kind) are full of sugar, such as glucose and fructose so that they can kick you out of ketosis.

- **Snacks:** Your favorite snacks such as donuts, cookies, cakes, and chocolate bars are strictly prohibited when you are following the ketogenic diet as they are loaded with a lot of sugar and trans-fat.

- **Grains:** Grains and starches are broken down into glucose; thus, they should be avoided at all costs. These include rice, oatmeal, rye, barley, wheat, corn, and basically, all types of grains imaginable.

- **Fruits:** Fruits contain high amounts of fructose. Fruits that contain high amounts of sugar include watermelon, bananas, and many others.

- **Root vegetables:** Root vegetables like sweet potatoes, potatoes, parsnips, and carrots contain high amounts of starch, which can be converted into simple sugar.

- **Processed oils:** Ketogenic diet advocates the consumption of healthy fats, but it discourages the consumption of processed oils such as vegetable oil, canola oil, corn oil, and soy oil.

- **Alcoholic beverages:** Alcoholic beverages such as beer are high in sugar; thus, it is bad for ketosis.

- **Beans and legumes:** Beans and legumes are high in starch; thus it is converted into glucose.

If you are enjoying this book, please let me know your thoughts by leaving a short review on Amazon. I will personally read it…Thank you! And Now, Getting started with tons of delicious recipes!

CHAPTER 18:

Breakfast Recipes

Buckwheat Spaghetti with Chicken Cabbage and Savory Food Recipes in Mass Sauce

Preparation Time: 15 minutes

Cooking time: 15 minutes'

Servings: 2

Ingredients:

For the noodles:

2-3 handfuls of cabbage leaves (removed from the stem and cut)

Buckwheat noodles 150g / 5oz (100% buckwheat, without wheat)

3-4 shiitake mushrooms, sliced

1 teaspoon of coconut oil or butter

1 brown onion, finely chopped

1 medium chicken breast, sliced or diced

1 long red pepper, thinly sliced (seeds in or out depending on how hot you like it)

2 large garlic cloves, diced

2-3 tablespoons of Tamari sauce (gluten-free soy sauce)

For the miso dressing:

1 tablespoon and a half of fresh organic miso

1 tablespoon of Tamari sauce

1 tablespoon of extra virgin olive oil

1 tablespoon of lemon or lime juice

1 teaspoon of sesame oil (optional)

Directions:

Boil a medium saucepan of water. Add the black cabbage and cook 1 minute, until it is wilted. Remove and reserve, but reserve the water and return to boiling. Add your soba noodles and cook according to the directions on the package (usually about 5 minutes). Rinse with cold water and reserve.

In the meantime, fry the shiitake mushrooms in a little butter or coconut oil (about a teaspoon) for 2-3 minutes, until its color is lightly browned on each side. Sprinkle with sea salt and reserve.

In that same pan, heat more coconut oil or lard over medium-high heat. Fry the onion and chili for 2-3 minutes, and then add the chicken pieces. Cook 5 minutes on medium heat, stirring a few times, then add the garlic, tamari sauce, and a little water. Cook for another 2-3 minutes, stirring continuously until your chicken is cooked.

Finally, add the cabbage and soba noodles and stir the chicken to warm it.

Stir the miso sauce and sprinkle the noodles at the end of the cooking, in this way you will keep alive all the beneficial probiotics in the miso.

Nutrition:

305 calories

Fat 11

Fiber 7

Carbs 9

Protein 12

Asian King Jumped Jamp

Preparation Time: 15 minutes

Cooking time: 10 minutes

Servings: 4

Ingredients:

150 g / 5 oz. of raw shelled prawns, not chopped

Two teaspoons of tamari (you can use soy sauce if you don't avoid gluten)

Two teaspoons of extra virgin olive oil

75 g / 2.6 oz. soba (buckwheat pasta)

1 garlic clove, finely chopped

1 bird's eye chili, finely chopped

1 teaspoon finely chopped fresh ginger.

20 g / 0.7 oz. of sliced red onions

40 g / 1.4 oz. of celery, cut and sliced

75 g / 2.6 oz. of chopped green beans

50 g / 1.7 oz. of chopped cabbage

100 ml / ½ cup of chicken broth

5 g celery or celery leaves

Directions:

Heat a pan over high heat, and then cook the prawns in 1 teaspoon of tamari and 1 teaspoon of oil for 2-3 minutes. Transfer the prawns to a plate. Clean the pan with kitchen paper as it will be reused.

Cook your noodles in boiling water for 5-8 minutes or as indicated on the package. Drain and set aside.

Meanwhile, fry the garlic, chili and ginger, red onion, celery, beans, and cabbage in the remaining oil over medium-high heat for 2-3 minutes. Add your broth and allow it to boil, and then simmer for a minute or two, until the vegetables are cooked but crunchy.

Add shrimp, noodles and celery/celery leaves to the pan, bring to a boil again, then remove from the heat and serve.

Nutrition:

Calories 223 Protein 34

Fat 2 Carbs 6

Buckwheat Pasta Salad

Preparation Time: 10 minutes

Cooking time: 30 minutes

Servings: 4

Ingredients:

50 g / 1.7 oz. buckwheat pasta

Large handful of rockets

A small handful of basil leaves

Eight cherry tomatoes halved

1/2 avocado, diced

Ten olives

1 tablespoon. extra olive virgin oil

20 g / 0.70 oz. pine nuts

Directions:

Combine all the Ingredients: except your pine nuts. Arrange your combination on a plate, and then scatter the pine nuts over the top.

Nutrition:

125 calories

Fat 6

Fiber 5

Carbs 10

Protein 11

Greek Salad Skewers

Preparation Time: 35 minutes

Cooking time: 0 minutes

Servings: 2

Ingredients:

Two wooden skewers, soaked in water for 30 minutes before use

Eight large black olives

Eight cherry tomatoes

1 yellow pepper, cut into eight squares.

½ red onions, you can cut in half and separated into eight pieces

100 g / 3.5 oz. (about 10cm) cucumber, cut into four slices and halved

100 g / 3.5 oz. feta, cut into eight cubes

For the dressing:

1 tablespoon. extra olive virgin oil

Juice of ½ lemons

1 teaspoon. of your balsamic vinegar

½ clove garlic, ensure it peeled and crushed

Basil leaves chopped (or ½ teaspoon. dried mixed herbs to replace basil and oregano)

Oregano leaves,

Salt and grounded black pepper

Directions:

Blend each skewer with the salad Ingredients: in the order

Put all your dressing Ingredients: into a bowl and mix thoroughly. Pour over the skewers.

Nutrition:

Calories 99 Protein 34

Fat 4 Carbs 5

Kale, Edamame and Tofu Curry

Preparation Time: 20 minutes

Cooking time: 40 minutes

Servings: 3

Ingredients:

1 tablespoon rapeseed oil

1 large onion, chopped

Four cloves garlic, peeled and grated

1 large thumb (7cm) fresh ginger, peeled and grated

1 red chili, deseeded and thinly sliced

1/2 teaspoon ground turmeric

1/4 teaspoon cayenne pepper

1 teaspoon paprika

1/2 teaspoon ground cumin

1 teaspoon salt

250 g / 9 oz. dried red lentils

1-liter boiling water

50 g / 1.7 oz. frozen soya beans

200 g / 7 oz. firm tofu, chopped into cubes

Two tomatoes, roughly chopped

Juice of 1 lime

200 g / 7 oz. kale leaves stalk removed and torn

Directions:

Put the oil in a pan over low heat. Add your onion and cook for 5 minutes before adding the garlic, ginger, and chili and cooking for a further 2 minutes. Add your turmeric, cayenne, paprika, cumin, and salt and Stir through before adding the red lentils and stirring again.

Pour in the boiling water and allow it to simmer for 10 minutes, reduce the heat and cook for about 20-30 minutes until the curry has a thick '•porridge' consistency.

Add your tomatoes, tofu and soya beans and cook for a further 5 minutes. Add your kale leaves and lime juice and cook until the kale is just tender.

Nutrition:

Calories 133

Carbohydrate 54

Protein 43

Chocolate Cupcakes with Matcha Icing

Preparation Time: 35 minutes

Cooking time: 0 minutes

Servings: 4

Ingredients:

150g / 5 oz. self-rising flour

200 g / 7 oz. caster sugar

60 g / 2.1 oz. cocoa

½ teaspoon. salt

½ teaspoon. fine espresso coffee, decaf if preferred

120 ml / ½ cup milk

½ teaspoon. vanilla extract

50 ml / ¼ cup vegetable oil

1 egg

120 ml / ½ cup of water

For the icing:

50 g / 1.7 oz. butter,

50 g / 1.7 oz. icing sugar

1 tablespoon matcha green tea powder

½ teaspoon vanilla bean paste

50 g / 1.7 oz. soft cream cheese

Directions:

Heat the oven and Line a cupcake tin with paper

Put the flour, sugar, cocoa, salt, and coffee powder in a large bowl and mix well.

Add milk, vanilla extract, vegetable oil, and egg to dry Ingredients: and use an electric mixer to beat until well combined. Gently pour the boiling water slowly and beat on low speed until completely combined. Use the high speed to beat for another minute to add air to the dough. The dough is much more liquid than a normal cake mix. Have faith; It will taste fantastic!

Arrange the dough evenly between the cake boxes. Each cake box must not be more than ¾ full. Bake for 15-18 minutes, until the dough resumes when hit. Remove from oven and allow cooling completely before icing.

To make the icing, beat your butter and icing sugar until they turn pale and smooth. Add the matcha powder and vanilla and mix again. Add the cream cheese and beat until it is smooth. Pipe or spread on the cakes.

Nutrition:

calories435

Fat 5

Fiber 3

Carbs 7

Protein 9

Sesame Chicken Salad

Preparation Time: 20 minutes

Cooking time: 0 minutes

Servings: 4

Ingredients:

1 tablespoon of sesame seeds

1 cucumber, peeled, halved lengthwise, without a teaspoon, and sliced.

100 g / 3.5 oz. cabbage, chopped

60 g pak choi, finely chopped

½ red onion, thinly sliced

Large parsley (20 g / 0.7 oz.), chopped.

150 g / 5 oz. cooked chicken, minced

For the dressing:

1 tablespoon of extra virgin olive oil

1 teaspoon of sesame oil

1 lime juice

1 teaspoon of light honey

2 teaspoons soy sauce

Directions:

Roast your sesame seeds in a dry pan for 2 minutes until they become slightly golden and fragrant.

Transfer to a plate to cool.

In a small bowl, mix olive oil, sesame oil, lime juice, honey, and soy sauce to prepare the dressing.

Place the cucumber, black cabbage, pak choi, red onion, and parsley in a large bowl and mix gently.

Pour over the dressing and mix again.

Distribute the salad between two dishes and complete with the shredded chicken. Sprinkle with sesame seeds just before serving.

Nutrition:

Calories 345

Fat 5

Fiber 2

Carbs 10

Protein 4

Bacon Appetizers

Preparation Time: 15 minutes

Cooking Time: 2 hours

Servings: 6

Ingredients:

1 pack Keto crackers

¾ cup Parmesan cheese, grated

1 lb. bacon, sliced thinly

Directions:

Preheat your oven to 250 degrees F.

Arrange the crackers on a baking sheet.

Sprinkle cheese on top of each cracker.

Wrap each cracker with the bacon.

Bake in the oven for 2 hours.

Nutrition:

Calories 440 Total Fat 33.4g

Saturated Fat 11g

Cholesterol 86mg

Sodium 1813mg

Total Carbohydrate 3.7g

Dietary Fiber 0.1g

Total Sugars 0.1g Protein 29.4g

Potassium 432mg

Antipasti Skewers

Preparation Time: 10 minutes

Cooking Time: 0 minute

Servings: 6

Ingredients:

6 small mozzarella balls

1 tablespoon olive oil

Salt to taste

1/8 teaspoon dried oregano

2 roasted yellow peppers, sliced into strips and rolled

6 cherry tomatoes

6 green olives, pitted

6 Kalamata olives pitted

2 artichoke hearts, sliced into wedges

6 slices salami, rolled

6 leaves fresh basil

Directions:

Toss the mozzarella balls in olive oil.

Season with salt and oregano.

Thread the mozzarella balls and the rest of the **Ingredients:** into skewers.

Serve in a platter.

Nutrition:

Calories 180

Total Fat 11.8g

Saturated Fat 4.5g

Cholesterol 26mg

Sodium 482mg

Total Carbohydrate 11.7g

Dietary Fiber 4.8g Total Sugars 4.1g

Protein 9.2g Potassium 538mg

Jalapeno Poppers

Preparation Time: 30 minutes

Cooking Time: 60 minutes

Servings: 10

Ingredients:

5 fresh jalapenos, sliced and seeded

4 oz. package cream cheese

¼ lb. bacon, sliced in half

Directions:

Preheat your oven to 275 degrees F.

Place a wire rack over your baking sheet.

Stuff each jalapeno with cream cheese and wrap in bacon.

Secure with a toothpick.

Place on the baking sheet.

Bake for 1 hour and 15 minutes.

Nutrition:

Calories 103

Total Fat 8.7g

Saturated Fat 4.1g

Cholesterol 25mg

Sodium 296mg

Total Carbohydrate 0.9g

Dietary Fiber 0.2g

Total Sugars 0.3g

Protein 5.2g

Potassium 93mg

BLT Party Bites

Preparation Time: 35 minutes

Cooking Time: 0 minute

Servings: 8

Ingredients:

4 oz. bacon, chopped

3 tablespoons panko breadcrumbs

1 tablespoon Parmesan cheese, grated

1 teaspoon mayonnaise

1 teaspoon lemon juice

Salt to taste

½ heart Romaine lettuce, shredded

6 cocktail tomatoes

Directions:

Put the bacon in a pan over medium heat.

Fry until crispy.

Transfer bacon to a plate lined with a paper towel.

Add breadcrumbs and cook until crunchy.

Transfer breadcrumbs to another plate, also lined with a paper towel.

Sprinkle Parmesan cheese on top of the breadcrumbs.

Mix the mayonnaise, salt and lemon juice.

Toss the Romaine in the mayo mixture.

Slice each tomato on the bottom to create a flat surface so it can stand by itself.

Slice the top off as well.

Scoop out the insides of the tomatoes.

Stuff each tomato with the bacon, Parmesan, breadcrumbs and top with the lettuce.

Nutrition:

Calories 107

Total Fat 6.5g

Saturated Fat 2.1g

Cholesterol 16mg

Sodium 360mg

Total Carbohydrate 5.4g

Dietary Fiber 1.5g

Total Sugars 3.3g

Protein 6.5g

Potassium 372mg

Eggs Benedict Deviled Eggs

Preparation Time: 15 minutes

Cooking Time: 25 minutes

Servings: 16

Ingredients:

8 hardboiled eggs, sliced in half

1 tablespoon lemon juice

½ teaspoon mustard powder

1 pack Hollandaise sauce mix, prepared according to the direction in the packaging

1 lb. asparagus, trimmed and steamed

4 oz. bacon, cooked and chopped

Directions:

Scoop out the egg yolks.

Mix the egg yolks with lemon juice, mustard powder and 1/3 cup of the Hollandaise sauce.

Spoon the egg yolk mixture into each of the egg whites.

Arrange the asparagus spears on a serving plate.

Top with the deviled eggs.

Sprinkle remaining sauce and bacon on top.

Nutrition:

Calories 80

Total Fat 5.3g

Saturated Fat 1.7g

Cholesterol 90mg

Sodium 223mg

Total Carbohydrate 2.1g

Dietary Fiber 0.6g

Total Sugars 0.7g

Protein 6.2g

Potassium 133mg

Spinach Meatballs

Preparation Time: 20 minutes

Cooking Time: 30 minutes

Servings: 4

Ingredients:

1 cup spinach, chopped

1 ½ lb. ground turkey breast

1 onion, chopped

3 cloves garlic, minced

1 egg, beaten

¼ cup milk

¾ cup breadcrumbs

½ cup Parmesan cheese, grated

Salt and pepper to taste

2 tablespoons butter

2 tablespoons Keto flour

10 oz. Italian cheese, shredded

½ teaspoon nutmeg, freshly grated

¼ cup parsley, chopped

Directions:

Preheat your oven to 400 degrees F.

Mix all the Ingredients: in a large bowl.

Form meatballs from the mixture.

Bake in the oven for 20 minutes.

Nutrition:

Calories 374

Total Fat 18.5g

Saturated Fat 10g

Cholesterol 118mg

Sodium 396mg

Total Carbohydrate 11.3g

Dietary Fiber 1g

Total Sugars 1.7g

Protein 34.2g

Potassium 336mg

Bacon-Wrapped Asparagus

Preparation Time: 10 minutes

Cooking Time: 20 minutes

Servings: 6

Ingredients:

1 ½ lb. asparagus spears, sliced in half

6 slices bacon

2 tablespoons olive oil

Salt and pepper to taste

Directions:

Preheat your oven to 400 degrees F.

Wrap a handful of asparagus with bacon.

Secure with a toothpick.

Drizzle with the olive oil.

Season with salt and pepper.

Bake in the oven for 20 minutes or until bacon is crispy.

Nutrition:

Calories 166

Total Fat 12.8g

Saturated Fat 3.3g

Cholesterol 21mg

Sodium 441mg

Total Carbohydrate 4.7g

Dietary Fiber 2.4g

Total Sugars 2.1g

Protein 9.5g

Potassium 337mg

Kale Chips

Preparation Time: 5 minutes

Cooking Time: 12 minutes

Servings: 2

Ingredients:

1 bunch kale, removed from the stems

2 tablespoons extra virgin olive oil

1 tablespoon garlic salt

Directions:

Preheat your oven to 350 degrees F.

Coat the kale with olive oil.

Arrange on a baking sheet.

Bake for 12 minutes.

Sprinkle with garlic salt.

Nutrition:

Calories 100

Total Fat 7g 9%

Saturated Fat 1g 5%

Cholesterol 0mg 0%

Sodium 30mg 1%

Total Carbohydrate 8.5g 3%

Dietary Fiber 1.2g 4%

Total Sugars 0.5g

Protein 2.4g

Calcium 92mg 7%

Iron 1mg 6%

Potassium 352mg

Bacon, Mozzarella & Avocado

Preparation Time: 15 minutes

Cooking Time: 15 minutes

Servings: 2

Ingredients:

3 slices bacon

1 cup mozzarella cheese, shredded

6 eggs, beaten

2 tablespoons butter

½ avocado

1 oz. cheddar cheese, shredded

Salt and pepper to taste

Directions:

Fry the bacon in a pan until crispy.

Transfer to a plate and set aside.

Place the mozzarella cheese the pan and cook until the edges have browned.

Cook the eggs in butter.

Stuff mozzarella with scrambled eggs, bacon and mashed avocado.

Sprinkle cheese on top.

Season with salt and pepper.

Nutrition:

Calories 645

Total Fat 53.6g

Saturated Fat 21.9g

Cholesterol 575mg

Sodium 1101mg

Total Carbohydrate 6.5g

Dietary Fiber 3.4g

Total Sugars 1.4g

Protein 35.8g

Potassium 600mg

Keto Cheese Chips

Preparation Time: 10 minutes

Cooking Time: 10 minutes

Servings: 3

Ingredients:

1 ½ cups cheddar cheese, shredded

3 tablespoons ground flaxseed meal

Garlic salt to taste

Directions:

Preheat your oven to 425 degrees F.

Create a small pile of 2 tablespoons cheddar cheese on a baking sheet.

Sprinkle flaxseed on top of each chip.

Season with garlic salt.

Bake in the oven for 10 minutes.

Let cool before serving.

Nutrition:

Calories 288

Total Fat 22.2g

Saturated Fat 11.9g

Cholesterol 59mg

Sodium 356mg

Total Carbohydrate 5.8g

Dietary Fiber 4g

Total Sugars 0.3g

Protein 17.1g

Potassium 57mg

Beef & Broccoli

Preparation Time: 10 minutes

Cooking Time: 15 minutes

Servings: 2

Ingredients:

¼ cup coconut amino, divided

1 teaspoon garlic, minced and divided

1 teaspoon fresh ginger, minced and divided

8 oz. beef, sliced thinly

1 ½ tablespoon avocado oil, divided

2 ½ cups broccolis, sliced into florets

¼ cup low sodium beef stock

½ teaspoon sesame oil

Salt to taste

Sesame seeds

Green onion, chopped

Directions:

In a bowl, mix the one tablespoon coconut amino with half of the ginger and garlic.

Marinate the beef into this mixture for 1 hour.

Cover with foil and place in the refrigerator.

Put 1 tablespoon oil in a pan over medium heat.

Add the broccoli and cook for 3 minutes.

Add the remaining ginger and garlic.

Cook for 1 minute.

Reduce heat.

Cover the pan with its lid.

Cook until the broccoli is tender but still a little crunchy.

Transfer the broccoli to a platter.

Increase the heat and add the remaining oil.

Add the beef and cook for 3 minutes.

Put the broccoli back.

In a bowl, mix the remaining coconut amino, broth and sesame oil.

Pour into the pan.

Cook until the sauce has thickened.

Season with salt.

Garnish with sesame seeds and green onion.

Nutrition:

Calories 298

Total Fat 10g

Saturated Fat 3.1g

Cholesterol 101mg

Sodium 1989mg

Total Carbohydrate 12.2g

Dietary Fiber 4g

Total Sugars 2.7g

Protein 40g

Potassium 958mg

Beef Stroganoff

Preparation Time: 20 minutes

Cooking Time: 2 hours and 10 minutes

Servings: 10

Ingredients:

¼ cup avocado oil

1 white onion, chopped

2 teaspoons garlic, minced

3 lb. beef brisket, fat trimmed and sliced into bite-size pieces

Salt and pepper to taste

2 teaspoons ground thyme

1 ½ cups beef broth

2 tablespoons apple cider vinegar

16 oz. fresh mushrooms, sliced

¾ cup sour cream

¼ cup mayonnaise

1 ½ teaspoon xanthan gum

Directions:

Place your pan over medium heat.

Add the oil, onion and garlic.

Sauté for 3 minutes.

Add the beef.

Season with salt, pepper and thyme.

Cook for 8 minutes, stirring frequently.

Reduce heat and add beef broth and vinegar.

Simmer for 30 minutes.

Add mushrooms and cover the pan.

Simmer for 1 hour and 30 minutes.

Remove the pan from the stove.

Stir in the mayonnaise and sour cream.

Gradually stir in the xanthan gum until the sauce has thickened.

Cover the pan and let sit for 10 minutes before serving.

Nutrition:

Calories 343 Total Fat 15.1g

Saturated Fat 6g

Cholesterol 131mg

Sodium 292mg   Total Carbohydrate 6.5g

Dietary Fiber 2g

Total Sugars 1.8g

Protein 44.4g

Potassium 789mg

Garlic Butter Steak

Preparation Time: 10 minutes

Cooking Time: 15 minutes

Servings: 2

Ingredients:

2 rib-eye steaks, trimmed

1 ½ tablespoons olive oil, divided

Salt and pepper to taste

2 tablespoons butter

2 cloves garlic, minced

2 sprigs fresh rosemary, chopped

Directions:

Dry the steaks using a paper towel.

Put a cast-iron skillet over high heat.

Wait until the skillet starts to smoke.

Add 1 tablespoon oil to the skillet.

Coat the steaks with the remaining oil.

Season steaks with salt and pepper.

Add the steaks to the hot pan.

Sear for 5 to 7 minutes for medium and up to 10 minutes for medium-well.

Reduce the heat to low.

Add the butter, garlic and rosemary.

Cook for another minute.

Let the steak rest before slicing and serving.

Nutrition:

Calories 547

Total Fat 48.1g

Saturated Fat 19.3g

Cholesterol 120mg

Sodium 142mg

Total Carbohydrate 1.2g

Dietary Fiber 0.4g

Total Sugars 0g

Protein 26.9g

Potassium 18mg

Beef Shawarma

Preparation Time: 5 minutes

Cooking Time: 15 minutes

Servings: 4

Ingredients:

2 tablespoons olive oil

1 lb. lean ground beef

1 cup onion, sliced

Salt to taste

3 tablespoons shawarma mix

3 cups cabbage, shredded

2 tablespoons water

1/4 cup parsley, chopped

Directions:

Put your pan over medium heat.

Once the pan starts to sizzle, add the olive oil.

Add the ground beef.

Add the onion and cook for 4 minutes.

Season with salt and shawarma mix.

Add the cabbage.

Pour in the water.

Cover the pan and steam for 1 minute.

Garnish with parsley before serving.

Nutrition:

Calories 330

Total Fat 15.3g

Saturated Fat 4.1g

Cholesterol 101mg

Sodium 201mg

Total Carbohydrate 12g

Dietary Fiber 4.3g

Total Sugars 2.9g

Protein 35.9g

Potassium 609mg

CHAPTER 19:

Lunch Recipes

Chicken, Bacon and Avocado Cloud Sandwiches

Preparation Time: 10 minutes

Cooking time: 25 minutes

Servings: 6

Ingredients:

For cloud bread

3 large eggs

4 oz. cream cheese

½ tablespoon. ground psyllium husk powder

½ teaspoon baking powder

A pinch of salt

To assemble sandwich

6 slices of bacon, cooked and chopped

6 slices pepper Jack cheese

½ avocado, sliced

1 cup cooked chicken breasts, shredded

3 tablespoons. mayonnaise

Directions:

Preheat your oven to 300 degrees.

Prepare a baking sheet by lining it with parchment paper.

Separate the egg whites and egg yolks, and place into separate bowls.

Whisk the egg whites until very stiff. Set aside.

Combined egg yolks and cream cheese.

Add the psyllium husk powder and baking powder to the egg yolk mixture. Gently fold in.

Add the egg whites into the egg mixture and gently fold in.

Dollop the mixture onto the prepared baking sheet to create 12 cloud bread. Use a spatula to spread the circles around to form ½-inch thick pieces gently.

Bake for 25 minutes or until the tops are golden brown.

Allow the cloud bread to cool completely before serving. It can be refrigerated for up to 3 days or frozen for up to 3 months. If food prepping, place a layer of parchment paper between each bread slice to avoid having them getting stuck together. Simply toast in the oven for 5 minutes when it is time to servings.

To assemble sandwiches, place mayonnaise on one side of one cloud bread. Layer with the remaining sandwich Ingredients: and top with another slice of cloud bread. Servings.

Nutrition:

Calories: 333 kcal

Carbs: 5g

Fat: 26g

Protein: 19.9g

Roasted Lemon Chicken Sandwich

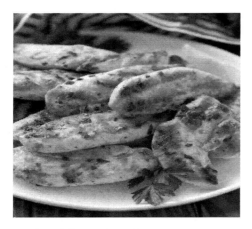

Preparation Time: 15 minutes

Cooking time: 1 hour 30 minutes

Servings: 12

Ingredients:

1 kg whole chicken

5 tablespoons. butter

1 lemon, cut into wedges

1 tablespoon. garlic powder

Salt and pepper to taste

2 tablespoons. mayonnaise

Keto-friendly bread

Directions:

Preheat the oven to 350 degrees F.

Grease a deep baking dish with butter.

Ensure that the chicken is patted dry and that the gizzards have been removed.

Combine the butter, garlic powder, salt and pepper.

Rub the entire chicken with it, including in the cavity.

Place the lemon and onion inside the chicken and place the chicken in the prepared baking dish.

Bake for about 1½ hours, depending on the size of the chicken.

Baste the chicken often with the drippings. If the drippings begin to dry, add water. The chicken is done when a thermometer insert it into the thickest part of the thigh, reads 165 degrees F or when the clear juices run when the thickest part of the thigh is pierced.

Allow the chicken to cool before slicing.

To assemble the sandwich, shred some of the breast meat and mix with the mayonnaise. Place the mixture between the two bread slices.

To save the chicken, refrigerated for up to 5 days or freeze for up to 1 month.

Nutrition:

Calories: 214 kcal Carbs: 1.6 g

Fat: 11.8 g Protein: 24.4 g.

Keto-Friendly Skillet Pepperoni Pizza

Preparation Time: 10 minutes

Cooking time: 6 minutes

Servings: 4

Ingredients:

For Crust

½ cup almond flour

½ teaspoon baking powder

8 large egg whites, whisked into stiff peaks

Salt and pepper to taste

Toppings

3 tablespoons. unsweetened tomato sauce

½ cup shredded cheddar cheese

½ cup pepperoni

Directions

Gently incorporate the almond flour into the egg whites. Ensure that no lumps remain.

Stir in the remaining crust ingredients.

Heat a nonstick skillet over medium heat. Spray with nonstick spray.

Pour the batter into the heated skillet to cover the bottom of the skillet.

Cover the skillet with a lid and cook the pizza crust to cook for about 4 minutes or until bubbles that appear on the top.

Flip the dough and add the toppings, starting with the tomato sauce and ending with the pepperoni

Cook the pizza for 2 more minutes.

Allow the pizza to cool slightly before serving.

It can be stored in the refrigerator for up to 5 days and frozen for up to 1 month.

Nutrition:

Calories: 175 kcal Carbs: 1.9 g

Fat: 12 g Protein: 14.3 g.

Cheesy Chicken Cauliflower

Preparation Time: 5 minutes

Cooking time: 10 minutes

Servings: 4

Ingredients:

2 cups cauliflower florets, chopped

½ cup red bell pepper, chopped

1 cup roasted chicken, shredded (Lunch Recipes: Roasted Lemon Chicken Sandwich)

¼ cup shredded cheddar cheese

1 tablespoon. butter

1 tablespoon. sour cream

Salt and pepper to taste

Directions:

Stir fry the cauliflower and peppers in the butter over medium heat until the veggies are tender.

Add the chicken and cook until the chicken is warmed through.

Add the remaining **Ingredients:** and stir until the cheese is melted.

Serve warm.

Nutrition:

Calories: 144 kcal Carbs: 4 g

Fat: 8.5 g Protein: 13.2 g.

Chicken Soup

Preparation Time: 10 minutes

Cooking time: 25 minutes

Servings: 6

Ingredients:

4 cups roasted chicken, shredded (Lunch Recipes: Roasted Lemon Chicken Sandwich)

2 tablespoons. butter

2 celery stalks, chopped

1 cup mushrooms, sliced

4 cups green cabbage, cut into strips

2 garlic cloves, minced

6 cups chicken broth

1 carrot, sliced

Salt and pepper to taste

1 tablespoon. garlic powder

1 tablespoon. onion powder

Directions:

Sauté the celery, mushrooms and garlic in the butter in a pot over medium heat for 4 minutes.

Add broth, carrots, garlic powder, onion powder, salt, and pepper.

Simmer for 10 minutes or until the vegetables are tender.

Add the chicken and cabbage and simmer for another 10 minutes or until the cabbage is tender.

Servings warm.

It can be refrigerated for up to 3 days or frozen for up to 1 month.

Nutrition:

Calories: 279 kcal Carbs: 7.5 g

Fat: 12.3 g Protein: 33.4 g.

1 hard-boiled egg, chopped

1 cup romaine lettuce, chopped

1 tablespoon. olive oil

1 tablespoon. apple cider vinegar

Salt and pepper to taste

Directions:

Create the dressing by mixing apple cider vinegar, oil, salt and pepper. Combine all the other ingredients: in a mixing bowl. Drizzle with the dressing and toss. Servings.

It can be refrigerated for up to 3 days.

Nutrition:

Calories: 220 kcal Carbs: 2.8 g

Fat: 16.7 g Protein: 14.8 g.

Chicken Avocado Salad

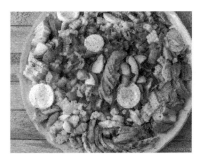

Preparation Time: 7 minutes

Cooking time: 10 minutes

Servings: 4

Ingredients:

1 cup roasted chicken, shredded (Lunch Recipes: Roasted Lemon Chicken Sandwich)

1 bacon strip, cooked and chopped

1/2 medium avocado, chopped

¼ cup cheddar cheese, grated

Chicken Broccoli Dinner

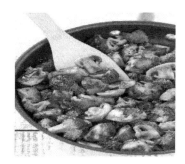

Preparation Time: 10 minutes

Cooking time: 5 minutes

Servings: 1

Ingredients:

1 roasted chicken leg (Lunch Recipes: Roasted Lemon Chicken Sandwich)

½ cup broccoli florets

½ tablespoon. unsalted butter softened

2 garlic cloves, minced

Salt and pepper to taste

Directions:

Boil the broccoli in lightly salted water for 5 minutes. Drain the water from the pot and keep the broccoli in the pool. Keep the lid on to keep the broccoli warm.

Mix all the butter, garlic, salt and pepper in a small bowl to create garlic butter.

Place the chicken, broccoli and garlic butter. Servings.

Nutrition:

Calories: 257 kcal Carbs: 5.1 g

Fat: 14 g Protein: 27.4 g.

Easy Meatballs

Preparation Time: 10 minutes

Cooking time: 20 minutes

 Servings: 4

Ingredients:

1 lb. ground beef

1 egg, beaten

Salt and pepper to taste

1 teaspoon garlic powder

1 teaspoon onion powder

2 tablespoons. butter

¼ cup mayonnaise

¼ cup pickled jalapeños

1 cup cheddar cheese, grated

Directions

Combine the cheese, mayonnaise, pickled jalapenos, salt, pepper, garlic powder and onion powder in a large mixing bowl.

Add the beef and egg and combine using clean hands.

Form large meatballs makes about 12.

Fry the meatballs in the butter over medium heat for about 4 minutes on each side or until golden brown.

Servings warm with a keto-friendly side.

The meatball mixture can also be used to make a meatloaf. Just preheat your oven to 400 degrees F, press the mixture into a loaf pan and bake for about 30 minutes or until the top is golden brown.

It can be refrigerated for up to 5 days or frozen for up to 3 months.

Nutrition:

Calories: 454 kcal Carbs: 5 g

Fat: 28.2 g Protein: 43.2 g.

Chicken Casserole

Preparation Time: 10 minutes

Cooking time: 40 minutes

Servings: 8

Ingredients:

1 lb. boneless chicken breasts, cut into 1" cubes

2 tablespoons. butter

4 tablespoons. green pesto

1 cup heavy whipping cream

¼ cup green bell peppers, diced

1 cup feta cheese, diced

1 garlic clove, minced

Salt and pepper to taste

Directions

Preheat your oven to 400 degrees F.

Season the chicken with salt and pepper, then batch fry in the butter until golden brown.

Place the fried chicken pieces in a baking dish. Add the feta cheese, garlic and bell peppers.

Combine the pesto and heavy cream in a bowl. Pour on top of the chicken mixture and spread with a spatula.

Bake for 30 minutes or until the casserole is light brown around the edges.

Servings warm.

It can be refrigerated for up to 5 days and frozen for 2 weeks.

Nutrition:

Calories: 294 kcal Carbs: 1.7 g

Fat: 22.7 g Protein: 20.1 g.

Lemon Baked Salmon

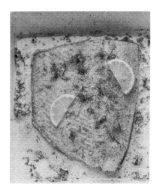

Preparation Time: 10 minutes

Cooking time: 30 minutes

Servings: 4

Ingredients:

1 lb. salmon

1 tablespoon. olive oil

Salt and pepper to taste

1 tablespoon. butter

1 lemon, thinly sliced

1 tablespoon. lemon juice

Directions:

Preheat your oven to 400 degrees F.

Grease a baking dish with the olive oil and place the salmon skin-side down.

Season the salmon with salt and pepper then top with the lemon slices.

Slice half the butter and place over the salmon.

Bake for 20minutes or until the salmon flakes easily. Melt the remaining butter in a saucepan. When it starts to bubble, remove from heat and allow to cool before adding the lemon juice.

Drizzle the lemon butter over the salmon and servings warm.

Nutrition:

Calories: 211 kcal

Carbs: 1.5 g

Fat: 13.5 g

Protein: 22.2 g.

Cauliflower Mash

Preparation Time: 10 minutes

Cooking time: 5 minutes

Servings: 8

Ingredients:

4 cups cauliflower florets, chopped

1 cup grated parmesan cheese

6 tablespoons. butter

½ lemon, juice and zest

Salt and pepper to taste

Directions:

Boil the cauliflower in lightly salted water over high heat for 5 minutes or until the florets are tender but still firm.

Strain the cauliflower in a colander and add the cauliflower to a food processor

Add the remaining Ingredients: and pulse the mixture to a smooth and creamy consistency

Servings with protein like salmon, chicken or meatballs.

It can be refrigerated for up to 3 days.

Nutrition:

Calories: 101 kcal

Carbs: 3.1 g

Fat: 9.5 g

Protein: 2.2 g.

Baked Salmon

Preparation Time: 10 minutes

Cooking Time: 10 minutes

Servings: 4

Ingredients:

Cooking spray

3 cloves garlic, minced

¼ cup butter

1 teaspoon lemon zest

2 tablespoons lemon juice

4 salmon fillets

Salt and pepper to taste

2 tablespoons parsley, chopped

Directions:

Preheat your oven to 425 degrees F.

Grease the pan with cooking spray.

In a bowl, mix the garlic, butter, lemon zest and lemon juice.

Sprinkle salt and pepper on salmon fillets.

Drizzle with the lemon butter sauce.

Bake in the oven for 12 minutes.

Garnish with parsley before serving.

Nutrition:

Calories 345

Total Fat 22.7g Saturated Fat 8.9g

Cholesterol 109mg Sodium 163mg

Total Carbohydrate 1.2g

Dietary Fiber 0.2g Total Sugars 0.2g

Protein 34.9g Potassium 718mg

Tuna Patties

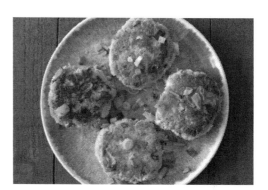

Preparation Time: 10 minutes

Cooking Time: 10 minutes

Servings: 8

Ingredients:

20 oz. canned tuna flakes

¼ cup almond flour

1 egg, beaten

2 tablespoons fresh dill, chopped

2 stalks green onion, chopped

Salt and pepper to taste

1 tablespoon lemon zest

¼ cup mayonnaise

1 tablespoon lemon juice

2 tablespoons avocado oil

Directions:

Combine all the Ingredients: except avocado oil, lemon juice and avocado oil in a large bowl.

Form 8 patties from the mixture.

In a pan over medium heat, add the oil.

Once the oil starts to sizzle, cook the tuna patties for 3 to 4 minutes per side.

Drain each patty on a paper towel.

Spread mayo on top and drizzle with lemon juice before serving.

Nutrition:

Calories 101

Total Fat 4.9g Saturated Fat 1.2g

Cholesterol 47mg Sodium 243mg

Total Carbohydrate 3.1g

Dietary Fiber 0.5g Total Sugars 0.7g

Protein 12.3g Potassium 60mg

Grilled Mahi Mahi with Lemon Butter Sauce

Preparation Time: 20 minutes

Cooking Time: 10 minutes

Servings: 6

Ingredients:

6 mahi mahi fillets

Salt and pepper to taste

2 tablespoons olive oil

6 tablespoons butter

¼ onion, minced

½ teaspoon garlic, minced

¼ cup chicken stock

1 tablespoon lemon juice

Directions:

Preheat your grill to medium heat.

Season fish fillets with salt and pepper.

Coat both sides with olive oil.

Grill for 3 to 4 minutes per side.

Place fish on a serving platter.

In a pan over medium heat, add the butter and let it melt.

Add the onion and sauté for 2 minutes.

Add the garlic and cook for 30 seconds.

Pour in the chicken stock.

Simmer until the stock has been reduced to half.

Add the lemon juice.

Pour the sauce over the grilled fish fillets.

Nutrition:

Calories 234

Total Fat 17.2g

Saturated Fat 8.3g

Cholesterol 117mg

Sodium 242mg

Total Carbohydrate 0.6g

Dietary Fiber 0.1g

Total Sugars 0.3g

Protein 19.1g

Potassium 385mg

Shrimp Scampi

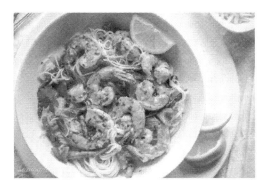

Preparation Time: 15 minutes

Cooking Time: 10 minutes

Servings: 6

Ingredients:

2 tablespoons olive oil

2 tablespoons butter

1 tablespoon garlic, minced

½ cup dry white wine

¼ teaspoon red pepper flakes

Salt and pepper to taste

2 lb. large shrimp, peeled and deveined

¼ cup fresh parsley, chopped

1 teaspoon lemon zest

2 tablespoons lemon juice

3 cups spaghetti squash, cooked

Directions:

In a pan over medium heat, add the oil and butter.

Cook the garlic for 2 minutes.

Pour in the wine.

Add the red pepper flakes, salt and pepper.

Cook for 2 minutes.

Add the shrimp.

Cook for 2 to 3 minutes.

Remove from the stove.

Add the parsley, lemon zest and lemon juice.

Serve on top of spaghetti squash.

Nutrition:

Calories 232

Total Fat 8.9g

Saturated Fat 3.2g

Cholesterol 226mg

Sodium 229mg

Total Carbohydrate 7.6g

Dietary Fiber 0.2g

Total Sugars 0.3g

Protein 28.9g

Potassium 104mg

CHAPTER 20:

Dinner Recipes

Beef-Stuffed Mushrooms

Preparation Time: 20 minutes

Cooking Time: 25 minutes

Servings: 4

Ingredients:

4 mushrooms, stemmed

3 tablespoons olive oil, divided

1 yellow onion, sliced thinly

1 red bell pepper, cut into strips

1 green bell pepper, cut into strips

Salt and pepper to taste

8 oz. beef, sliced thinly

3 oz. provolone cheese, sliced

Chopped parsley

Directions:

Preheat your oven to 350 degrees F.

Arrange the mushrooms on a baking pan.

Brush with oil.

Add the remaining oil to a pan over medium heat.

Cook onion and bell peppers for 5 minutes.

Season with salt and pepper.

Place onion mixture on a plate.

Cook the beef in the pan for 5 minutes.

Sprinkle with salt and pepper.

Add the onion mixture back to the pan.

Mix well.

Fill the mushrooms with the beef mixture and cheese.

Bake in the oven for 15 minutes.

Nutrition:

Calories 333 Total Fat 20.3 g

Saturated Fat 6.7 g Cholesterol 61 mg

Sodium 378 mg

Total Carbohydrate 8.2 g

Dietary Fiber 3.7 g Protein 25.2 g

Total Sugars 7 g Potassium 789 mg

Rib Roast

Preparation Time: 15 minutes

Cooking Time: 3 hours

Servings: 8

Ingredients:

1 rib roast

Salt to taste

12 cloves garlic, chopped

2 teaspoons lemon zest

6 tablespoons fresh rosemary, chopped

5 sprigs thyme

Directions:

Preheat your oven to 325 degrees F.

Season all sides of the rib roast with salt.

Place the rib roast in a baking pan.

Sprinkle with garlic, lemon zest and rosemary.

Add herb sprigs on top.

Roast for 3 hours.

Let rest for a few minutes and then slice and serve.

Nutrition:

Calories 329 Total Fat 27 g

Saturated Fat 9 g Cholesterol 59 mg

Sodium 498 mg Total Carbohydrate 5.3 g

Dietary Fiber 1.8 g Protein 18 g

Total Sugars 2 g

Potassium 493 mg

Beef Stir Fry

Preparation Time: 15 minutes

Cooking Time: 10 minutes

Servings: 4

Ingredients:

1 tablespoon soy sauce

1 tablespoon ginger, minced

1 teaspoon cornstarch

1 teaspoon dry sherry

12 oz. beef, sliced into strips

1 teaspoon toasted sesame oil

2 tablespoons oyster sauce

1 lb. baby bok choy, sliced

3 tablespoons chicken broth

Directions:

Mix soy sauce, ginger, cornstarch and dry sherry in a bowl.

Toss the beef in the mixture.

Pour oil into a pan over medium heat.

Cook the beef for 5 minutes, stirring.

Add oyster sauce, bok choy and chicken broth to the pan.

Cook for 1 minute.

Nutrition:

Calories 247 Total Fat 15.8 g

Saturated Fat 4 g Cholesterol 69 mg

Sodium 569 mg Total Carbohydrate 6.3 g

Dietary Fiber 1.1 g Protein 25 g

Sweet & Sour Pork

Preparation Time: 15 minutes

Cooking Time: 15 minutes

Servings: 4

Ingredients:

1 lb. pork chops - Salt and pepper to taste

½ cup sesame seeds - 2 tablespoons peanut oil

2 tablespoons soy sauce

3 tablespoons apricot jam

Chopped scallions

Directions:

Season pork chops with salt and pepper.

Press sesame seeds on both sides of pork.

Pour oil into a pan over medium heat.

Cook pork for 3 to 5 minutes per side.

Transfer to a plate.

In a bowl, mix soy sauce and apricot jam.

Simmer for 3 minutes.

Pour sauce over the pork and garnish with scallions before serving.

Nutrition:

Calories 414

Total Fat 27.5 g

Saturated Fat 5.6 g

Cholesterol 68 mg

Sodium 607 mg

Total Carbohydrate 12.9 g

Dietary Fiber 1.8 g

Protein 29 g

Total Sugars 9 g

Potassium 332 mg

Grilled Pork with Salsa

Preparation Time: 30 minutes

Cooking Time: 15 minutes

Servings: 4

Ingredients:

Salsa

1 onion, chopped

1 tomato, chopped

1 peach, chopped

1 apricot, chopped

1 tablespoon olive oil

1 tablespoon lime juice

2 tablespoons fresh cilantro, chopped

Salt and pepper to taste

Pork

1 lb. pork tenderloin, sliced

1 tablespoon olive oil

Salt and pepper to taste

½ teaspoon ground cumin

¾ teaspoon chili powder

Directions:

Combine salsa Ingredients: in a bowl.

Cover and refrigerate.

Brush pork tenderloin with oil.

Season with salt, pepper, cumin and chili powder.

Grill pork for 5 to 7 minutes per side.

Slice pork and serve with salsa.

Nutrition:

Calories 219

Total Fat 9.5 g

Saturated Fat 1.8 g

Cholesterol 74 mg

Sodium 512 mg

Total Carbohydrate 8.3 g

Dietary Fiber 1.5 g

Protein 24 g

Total Sugars 6 g

Potassium 600 mg

Garlic Pork Loin

Preparation Time: 15 minutes

Cooking Time: 1 hour

Servings: 6

Ingredients:

1 ½ lb. pork loin roast

4 cloves garlic, sliced into slivers

Salt and pepper to taste

Directions:

Preheat your oven to 425 degrees F.

Make several slits all over the pork roast.

Insert garlic slivers.

Sprinkle with salt and pepper.

Roast in the oven for 1 hour.

Nutrition:

Calories 235

Total Fat 13.3 g

Saturated Fat 2.6 g

Cholesterol 71 mg

Sodium 450 mg

Total Carbohydrate 1.7 g

Dietary Fiber 0.3 g

Protein 25.7 g

Total Sugars 3 g

Potassium 383 mg

Chicken Pesto

Preparation Time: 15 minutes

Cooking Time: 25 minutes

Servings: 4

Ingredients:

1 lb. chicken cutlet - Salt and pepper to taste

1 tablespoon olive oil - ½ cup onion, chopped

½ cup heavy cream - ½ cup dry white wine

1 tomato, chopped - ¼ cup pesto

2 tablespoons basil, chopped

Directions:

Season chicken with salt and pepper.

Pour oil into a pan over medium heat.

Cook chicken for 3 to 4 minutes per side.

Place the chicken on a plate.

Add the onion to the pan.

Cook for 1 minute.

Stir in the rest of the ingredients.

Bring to a boil.

Simmer for 15 minutes.

Put the chicken back to the pan.

Cook for 2 more minutes and then serve.

Nutrition:

Calories 371 Total Fat 23.7 g

Saturated Fat 9.2 g Cholesterol 117 mg

Sodium 361 mg Total Carbohydrate 5.7 g

Dietary Fiber 1 g

Protein 27.7 g

Total Sugars 3 g

Potassium 567 mg

Garlic Parmesan Chicken Wings

Preparation Time: 20 minutes

Cooking Time: 20 minutes

Servings: 8

Ingredients:

Cooking spray

½ cup all-purpose flour

Pepper to taste

2 tablespoons garlic powder

3 eggs, beaten

1 ¼ cups Parmesan cheese, grated

2 cups breadcrumbs

2 lb. chicken wings

Directions:

Preheat your oven to 450 degrees F.

Spray baking pan with oil.

In a bowl, mix the flour, pepper and garlic powder.

Add eggs to another bowl.

Mix the Parmesan cheese and breadcrumbs in another bowl.

Dip the chicken wings in the first, second and third bowls.

Spray chicken wings with oil.

Bake in the oven for 20 minutes.

Nutrition:

Calories 221

Total Fat 11.6 g

Saturated Fat 3.9 g

Cholesterol 122 mg

Sodium 242 mg

Total Carbohydrate 8 g

Dietary Fiber 0.4 g

Protein 16 g

Total Sugars 3 g

Potassium 163 mg

Crispy Baked Shrimp

Preparation Time: 15 minutes

Cooking Time: 10 minutes

Servings: 4

Ingredients:

¼ cup whole-wheat breadcrumbs

3 tablespoons olive oil, divided

1 ½ lb. jumbo shrimp, peeled and deveined

Salt and pepper to taste

2 tablespoons lemon juice

1 tablespoon garlic, chopped

2 tablespoons butter

¼ cup Parmesan cheese, grated

2 tablespoons chives, chopped

Directions:

Preheat your oven to 425 degrees F.

Add breadcrumbs to a pan over medium heat.

Cook until toasted.

Transfer to a plate.

Coat baking pan with 1 tablespoon oil.

Arrange shrimp in a single layer in a baking pan.

Season with salt and pepper.

Mix lemon juice, garlic and butter in a bowl.

Pour mixture on top of the shrimp.

Add Parmesan cheese and chives to the breadcrumbs.

Sprinkle breadcrumbs on top of the shrimp.

Bake for 10 minutes.

Nutrition:

Calories 340

Total Fat 18.7 g

Saturated Fat 6 g

Cholesterol 293 mg

Sodium 374 mg

Total Carbohydrate 6 g

Dietary Fiber 0.8 g

Protein 36.9 g

Total Sugars 2 g

Potassium 483 mg

Herbed Mediterranean Fish Fillet

Preparation Time: 20 minutes

Cooking Time: 1 hour

Servings: 6

Ingredients:

3 lb. sea bass fillet

Salt to taste

2 tablespoons tarragon, chopped

¼ cup dry white wine

3 tablespoons olive oil, divided

1 tablespoon butter

2 cloves garlic, minced

2 cups whole-wheat breadcrumbs

3 tablespoons parsley, chopped

3 tablespoons oregano, chopped

3 tablespoons fresh basil, chopped

Directions:

Preheat your oven to 350 degrees F.

Season fish with salt and tarragon.

Pour half of the oil into a roasting pan.

Stir in wine.

Add the fish in the roasting pan.

Bake in the oven for 50 minutes.

Add remaining oil to a pan over medium heat.

Cook herbs, breadcrumbs and salt.

Spread breadcrumb mixture on top of fish and bake for 5 minutes.

Nutrition:

Calories 288

Total Fat 12.7 g

Saturated Fat 2.9 g

Cholesterol 65 mg

Sodium 499 mg

Total Carbohydrate 10.4 g

Dietary Fiber 1.8 g

Protein 29.5 g

Total Sugars 1 g

Potassium 401 mg

Mushroom Stuffed with Ricotta

Preparation Time: 10 minutes

Cooking Time: 10 minutes

Servings: 4

Ingredients:

4 large mushrooms, stemmed

1 tablespoon olive oil

Salt and pepper to taste

¼ cup basil, chopped

1 cup ricotta cheese

¼ cup Parmesan cheese, grated

Directions:

Preheat your grill.

Coat the mushrooms with oil.

Season with salt and pepper.

Grill for 5 minutes.

Stuff each mushroom with a mixture of basil, ricotta cheese and Parmesan cheese.

Grill for another 5 minutes.

Nutrition:

Calories 259

Total Fat 17.3 g

Saturated Fat 5.4 g

Cholesterol 24 mg

Sodium 509 mg

Total Carbohydrate 14.9 g

Dietary Fiber 2.6 g

Protein 12.2 g

Total Sugars 7 g

Potassium 572 mg

Thai Chopped Salad

Preparation Time: 15 minutes

Cooking Time: 0 minutes

Servings: 4

Ingredients:

10 oz. kale and cabbage mix

14 oz. tofu, sliced into cubes and fried crispy

½ cup vinaigrette

Directions:

Arrange kale and cabbage in a serving platter.

Top with the tofu cubes.

Drizzle with the vinaigrette.

Nutrition:

Calories 332

Total Fat 15 g

Saturated Fat 1.5 g

Cholesterol 0 mg

Sodium 236 mg

Total Carbohydrate 26.3 g

Dietary Fiber 7.6 g

Protein 1.3 g

Total Sugars 13 g

Potassium 41 mg

Lemon & Rosema

ry Salmon

Preparation Time: 10 minutes

Cooking Time: 15 minutes

Servings: 4

Ingredients:

4 salmon fillets

Salt and pepper to taste

4 tablespoons butter

1 lemon, sliced

8 rosemary sprigs

Directions:

Season salmon with salt and pepper.

Place salmon on a foil sheet.

Top with butter, lemon slices and rosemary sprigs.

Fold the foil and seal.

Bake in the oven at 450 degrees F for 15 minutes.

Nutrition:

Calories 365

Total Fat 22 g

Saturated Fat 6 g

Cholesterol 86 mg

Sodium 445 mg

Total Carbohydrate 5 g

Dietary Fiber 1.9 g

Protein 29.8 g

Total Sugars 3 g

Potassium 782 mg

Chicken Kurma

Preparation Time: 20 minutes

Cooking Time: 25 minutes

Servings: 6

Ingredients:

1 tablespoon olive oil

1 onion, diced - 3 cloves garlic, sliced thinly

1 ginger, minced

2 tomatoes, diced

1 serrano pepper, minced

Salt and pepper to taste

1 teaspoon ground turmeric

1 tablespoon tomato paste

1 ½ lb. chicken, sliced

1 red bell pepper, chopped

Directions:

Pour oil into a pan over medium heat. Cook onion for 3 minutes. Add garlic, ginger, tomatoes, Serrano pepper, salt, pepper, turmeric and tomato paste. Bring to a boil.

Reduce heat and simmer for 10 minutes.

Add chicken and cook for 5 minutes.

Stir in red bell pepper.

Cook for 5 minutes.

Nutrition:

Calories 175 Total Fat 15.2 g

Saturated Fat 3 g Cholesterol 115 mg

Sodium 400 mg Total Carbohydrate 7 g

Dietary Fiber 1.8 g Protein 24 g

Total Sugars 3 g

Potassium 436 mg

Baked Lemon & Pepper Chicken

Preparation Time: 20 minutes

Cooking Time: 25 minutes

Servings: 4

Ingredients:

4 chicken breast fillets

Salt to taste

1 tablespoon olive oil

1 lemon, sliced thinly

1 tablespoon maple syrup

2 tablespoons lemon juice

2 tablespoons butter

Pepper to taste

Directions:

Preheat your oven to 425 degrees F.

Season chicken with salt.

Pour oil into a pan over medium heat.

Cook chicken for 5 minutes per side.

Transfer chicken to a baking pan.

Surround the chicken with the lemon slices.

Bake in the oven for 10 minutes.

Pour in maple syrup and lemon juice to the pan.

Put the butter on top of the chicken.

Sprinkle with pepper.

Bake for another 5 minutes.

Nutrition:

Calories 286

Total Fat 13 g

Saturated Fat 5 g

Cholesterol 109 mg

Sodium 448 mg

Total Carbohydrate 7 g

Dietary Fiber 1.4 g

Protein 34.8 g

Total Sugars 3 g

Potassium 350 mg

Skillet Chicken with White Wine Sauce

Preparation time: 5 minutes

Cooking time: 30 minutes

Servings: 4

Ingredients:

4 boneless chicken thighs

1 tsp. garlic powder

1 tsp. dried thyme

1 tbsp. olive oil

1 tbsp. butter

1 yellow onion diced

3 garlic cloves minced

1 cup dry white wine

½ cup heavy cream

fresh chopped parsley

salt and pepper

Directions:

Heat your oil in a skillet. Season your chicken, add it to the skillet, and then cook it about 5-7 mins.

Flip the chicken and cook until looking golden brown.

Remove the chicken to a plate.

Add butter to the skillet. Then add onions and cook them until softened.

Stir in garlic, salt and pepper, add the wine and cook for 4-5 mins.

Stir in the thyme and the heavy cream.

Place the breasts back to the skillet and leave to simmer for 2-3 mins. Top them with the parsley.

Nutrition:

Calories: 276 kcal Fats: 21 g

Carbs: 6 g Protein: 25 g

Stir Fry Kimchi and Pork Belly

Preparation time: 10 minutes

Cooking time: 18 minutes

Servings: 3

Ingredients:

300 g pork belly

1 lb. kimchi

1 tbsp. soy sauce

1 tbsp. rice wine

1 tbsp. sesame seeds

1 stalk green onion

Directions:

Slice the pork as thin as possible and marinate it in soy sauce and rice wine for 8-10 mins.

Heat a pan. When very hot, add the pork belly and stir-fry until brown.

Add the kimchi to the pan and stir-fry for 2 mins to let the flavors thoroughly mix.

Turn off heat and slice the green onion. Top with sesame seeds.

Nutrition:

Calories: 790 kcal Fats: 68 g

Carbs: 7 g Protein: 14 g

Lemon Butter Sauce with Fish

Preparation time: 10 minutes

Cooking time: 10 minutes

Servings: 2

Ingredients:

150 g thin white fish fillets

4 tbsps. butter

2 tbsps. white flour

2 tbsps. olive oil

1 tbsp. fresh lemon juice

salt and pepper

chopped parsley

Directions:

Place the butter in a small skillet over medium heat. Melt it and leave it, just stirring it casually. After 3 mins, pour into a small bowl.

Add lemon juice and season it, and set it aside.

Dry the fish with paper towels, season it to taste, and sprinkle with flour.

Heat oil in a skillet over high heat: when shimmering, add the fish and cook around 2-3 mins.

Remove to a plate and serve with the sauce. Top with parsley.

Nutrition:

Calories: 371 kcal

Fats: 27 g

Carbs: 3 g

Protein: 30 g

Pressure Cooker Crack Chicken

Preparation time: 5 minutes

Cooking time: 25 minutes

Servings: 8

Ingredients:

2 lbs. boneless chicken thighs.

2 slices bacon

8 ozs. cream cheese

1 scallion sliced

½ cup shredded cheddar

1 ½ tsp. garlic and onion powder

1 tsp. red pepper flakes and dried dill

salt and pepper

2 tbsps. apple cider vinegar

1 tbsp. dried chives

Directions:

On pressure cooker, use sauté mode and wait for it to heat up. Add the bacon and cook until crispy. Then set aside on a plate.

Add everything in the pot, except the cheddar cheese. On Manual high, pressure cooks them for 15 mins and then release it.

On a large plate, shred the chicken and then return to the pot and the cheddar.

Top with the bacon and scallion.

Nutrition:

Calories: 437 kcal

Fats: 28 g

Carbs: 5 g

Protein: 41 g

Bacon Bleu Cheese Filled Eggs

Preparation time: 10 minutes

Cooking time: 90-120 minutes

Servings: 3

Ingredients:

8 eggs

¼ cup crumbled bleu cheese

3 slices of cooked bacon

¼ cup sour cream

1/3 cup mayo

¼ tsp. pepper and dill

½ tsp. salt

1 tbsp. mustard

parsley

Directions:

Hard boil your eggs and then cut them half. Place the yolks in a bowl.

With a fork, mash the yolks, add the sour cream, mayo, bleu cheese, mustard, and the seasoning and mix until creamy enough for your taste. Slice up the bacon to small pieces. Stir in the rest of the **Ingredients:** and fill up the eggs.

Nutrition:

Calories: 217 kcal

Fats: 16 g

Carbs: 1 g

Protein: 6 g

Spinach Stuffed Chicken Breasts

Preparation time: 25 minutes

Cooking time: 15 minutes

Servings: 4

Ingredients:

1 ½ lb. chicken breasts

4 ozs. cream cheese

¼ cup frozen spinach

½ cup mozzarella

4 oz. artichoke hearts

¼ cup Greek yogurt

salt and pepper

2 tbsps. olive oil

Directions:

Pound the breasts about 1 inch thick. Cut each chicken down the middle, but don't cut through it. Make a pocket for the filling: Season the chicken.

In a bowl, combine the Greek yogurt, mozzarella, cream cheese, artichoke, and spinach. Next, season it. Mix until well-combined.

Fill all breasts equally with your mixture.

In a skillet over medium heat, add the oil and place your chicken. Cover the skillet and cook for 5-6 mins, turning the heat up in the last 1-2 mins.

Nutrition:

Calories: 288 kcal

Fats: 18 g

Carbs: 3 g

Protein: 31 g

Chicken with Lemon and Garlic

Preparation time: 5 minutes

Cooking time: 20 minutes

Servings: 4

Ingredients:

4 boneless chicken thighs

2 garlic cloves minced

Juice of 1 lemon

¼ tsp. smoked paprika, red chili flakes, garlic powder

2 tsp. Italian seasoning

1 tbsp. heavy cream

fresh parsley

¼ small onion

1 tbsp. olive oil

1½ tbsp. butter

salt and pepper

Directions:

Season your chicken with all spices.

In a skillet over medium heat, add the olive oil and cook for 5-6 mins on each side. Set aside on a plate.

Heat the skillet again and add in the butter. Stir in onion and garlic and add your lemon juice. Season them with everything left. After that, stir in your heavy cream. Once the sauce has thickened up, add the chicken back to the pot.

Serve it with lemon slices.

Nutrition:

Calories: 279 kcal Fats: 15 g

Carbs: 3 g Protein: 15 g

Chicken Pot Pie in a Slow Cooker

Preparation time: 3 hours

Cooking time: 35 minutes

Servings: 6

Ingredients:

For the filling:

1 cup chicken broth

¾ cup heavy whipping cream

3 ½ ozs. cooked chicken

½ cup mixed veggies

¼ onion

2 garlic cloves

salt and pepper

¼ tsp. rosemary

1 tsp. poultry seasoning

For the crust:

4 eggs

4 ½ tbsps. butter

1/3 cup coconut flour

1 1/3 cup shredded cheddar

2 tsp. full-fat sour cream

¼ tsp. baking powder

Directions:

Cook 1-1 ½ lbs. Chicken in the slow cooker for 3 hours on high.

Preheat your oven to 400°F.

Sauté your onion, veggies, garlic cloves and season with 2 tbsp. Butter in a skillet for 5-6 mins.

Add in the whipping cream, chicken broth, poultry, thyme, and rosemary.

Simmer them covered for 5 mins and don't forget to use a lot of liquid; otherwise, it will be scorched. Add the diced chicken, too.

Make the breading by mixing melted butter, salt, sour cream, and eggs before whisking them.

Add coconut flour and baking powder and stir until well-combined.

Stir in the cheddar cheese.

Bake in a 400°F oven for 15-20 mins.

Set oven to broil and move the pie to the top shelf. Broil for 2-4 mins to brown nicely.

Nutrition:

Calories: 301 kcal Carbs: 5 g

Protein: 15 g Fats: 24 g

Cheese Cauli Breadsticks

Preparation time: 10 minutes

Cooking time: 35 minutes

Servings: 6

Ingredients:

4 eggs

4 cups cauli

3 cups mozzarella cheese

4 cloves garlic

3 tsps. oregano

salt and pepper

Directions:

Preheat your oven 425°F. Prepare one baking sheet with paper on it.

Chop your cauli to florets. Add them to a food processor and then pulse.

Microwave it for 10 mins and then let it cool afterward. In a large bowl, add in the cauli, eggs,

2 cups of cheese, oregano, garlic and season it while mixing it.

Place the mixture on your sheet while forming your desired shape. Bake it for 20-25 mins. Finally, top it with the rest of the cheese and bake for another 5 mins until golden and well melted.

Nutrition:

Calories: 185 kcal

Carbs: 4g

Protein: 11 g

Fats: 12 g

CHAPTER 21:

Soup and Stew Recipes

Winter Comfort stew

Cooking Time: 50 minutes

Preparation Time: 15 minutes

Servings: 6

Ingredients:

2 tbsp. olive oil

1 small yellow onion, chopped

2 garlic cloves, chopped

2 lb. grass-fed beef chuck, cut into 1-inch cubes

1 (14-oz.) can sugar-free crushed tomatoes

2 tsp. ground allspice

1½ tsp. red pepper flakes

½ C. homemade beef broth

6 oz. green olives pitted

8 oz. fresh baby spinach

2 tbsp. fresh lemon juice

Salt and freshly ground black pepper, to taste

¼ C. fresh cilantro, chopped

Directions:

In a pan, heat the oil in a pan over high heat and sauté the onion and garlic for about 2-3 minutes.

Add the beef and cook for about 3-4 minutes or until browned, stirring frequently.

Add the tomatoes, spices and broth and bring to a boil.

Reduce the heat to low and simmer, covered for about 30-40 minutes or until the desired doneness of the beef.

Stir in the olives and spinach and simmer for about 2-3 minutes.

Stir in the lemon juice, salt and black pepper and remove from the heat.

Serve hot with the garnishing of cilantro.

Nutrition:

Calories: 388

Carbohydrates: 8g

Protein: 485g

Fat: 17.7g

Sugar: 2.6g

Sodium: 473mg

Fiber: 3.1g

Ideal Cold Weather Stew

Cooking Time: 2 hours 40 minutes

Preparation Time: 20 minutes

Servings: 6

Ingredients:

3 tbsp. olive oil, divided

8 oz. fresh mushrooms, quartered

1¼ lb. grass-fed beef chuck roast, trimmed and cubed into 1-inch size

2 tbsp. tomato paste

½ tsp. dried thyme

1 bay leaf

5 C. homemade beef broth

6 oz. celery root, peeled and cubed

4 oz. yellow onions, chopped roughly

3 oz. carrot, peeled and sliced

2 garlic cloves, sliced

Salt and freshly ground black pepper, to taste

Directions:

In a Dutch oven, heat 1 tbsp. Of the oil over medium heat and cook the mushrooms for about 2 minutes, without stirring.

Stir the mushroom and cook for about 2 minutes more.

With a slotted spoon, transfer the mushroom onto a plate.

In the same pan, heat the remaining oil over medium-high heat and sear the beef cubes for about 4-5 minutes.

Stir in the tomato paste, thyme and bay leaf and cook for about 1 minute.

Stir in the broth and bring to a boil.

Reduce the heat to low and simmer, covered for about 1½ hours.

Stir in the mushrooms, celery, onion, carrot and garlic and simmers for about 40-60 minutes.

Stir in the salt and black pepper and remove from the heat.

Serve hot.

Nutrition:

Calories: 447 Carbohydrates: 7.4g

Protein: 30.8g Fat: 32.3g

Sugar: 8g Sodium: 764mg Fiber: 1.9g

Weekend Dinner Stew

Cooking Time: 55 minutes

Preparation Time: 15 minutes

Servings: 6

Ingredients:

1½ lb. grass-fed beef stew meat, trimmed and cubed into 1-inch size

Salt and freshly ground black pepper, to taste

1 tbsp. olive oil

1 C. homemade tomato puree

4 C. homemade beef broth

2 C. zucchini, chopped

2 celery ribs, sliced

½ C. carrots, peeled and sliced

2 garlic cloves, minced

½ tbsp. dried thyme

1 tsp. dried parsley

1 tsp. dried rosemary

1 tbsp. paprika

1 tsp. onion powder

1 tsp. garlic powder

Directions:

In a large bowl, add the beef cubes, salt and black pepper and toss to coat well.

In a large pan, heat the oil over medium-high heat and cook the beef cubes for about 4-5 minutes or until browned.

Add the remaining **Ingredients:** and stir to combine.

Increase the heat to high and bring to a boil.

Reduce the heat to low and simmer, covered for about 40-50 minutes.

Stir in the salt and black pepper and remove from the heat.

Serve hot.

Nutrition:

Calories: 293 Carbohydrates: 8g

Protein: 9.3g Fat: 10.7g

Sugar: 4g Sodium: 223mg Fiber: 2.3g

Mexican Pork Stew

Cooking Time: 2 hours 10 minutes

Preparation Time: 15 minutes

Servings: 1

Ingredients:

3 tbsp. unsalted butter

2½ lb. boneless pork ribs, cut into ¾-inch cubes

1 large yellow onion, chopped

4 garlic cloves, crushed

1½ C. homemade chicken broth

2 (10-oz.) cans sugar-free diced tomatoes

1 C. canned roasted poblano chiles

2 tsp. dried oregano

1 tsp. ground cumin

Salt, to taste

¼ C. fresh cilantro, chopped

2 tbsp. fresh lime juice

Directions:

In a large pan, melt the butter over medium-high heat and cook the pork, onions and garlic for about 5 minutes or until browned.

Add the broth and scrape up the browned bits.

Add the tomatoes, poblano chiles, oregano, cumin, and salt and bring to a boil.

Reduce the heat to medium-low and simmer, covered for about 2 hours.

Stir in the fresh cilantro and lime juice and remove from heat.

Serve hot.

Nutrition:

Calories: 288 Carbohydrates: 8.8g

Protein: 39.6g Fat: 10.1g Sugar: 4g

Sodium: 283mg Fiber: 2.8g

Hungarian Pork Stew

Cooking Time: 2 hours 20 minutes

Preparation Time: 15 minutes

Servings: 10

Ingredients:

3 tbsp. olive oil

3½ lb. pork shoulder, cut into 4 portions

1 tbsp. butter

2 medium onions, chopped

16 oz. tomatoes, crushed

5 garlic cloves, crushed

2 Hungarian wax peppers, chopped

3 tbsp. Hungarian Sweet paprika

1 tbsp. smoked paprika

1 tsp. hot paprika

½ tsp. caraway seeds

1 bay leaf

1 C. homemade chicken broth

1 packet unflavored gelatin

2 tbsp. fresh lemon juice

Pinch of xanthan gum

Salt and freshly ground black pepper, to taste

Directions:

In a heavy-bottomed pan, heat 1 tbsp. Of oil over high heat and sear the pork for about 2-3 minutes or until browned.

Transfer the pork onto a plate and cut it into bite-sized pieces.

In the same pan, heat 1 tbsp. of oil and butter over medium-low heat and sauté the onions for about 5-6 minutes.

With a slotted spoon, transfer the onion into a bowl. In the same pan, add the tomatoes and cook for about 3-4 minutes, without stirring.

Meanwhile, in a small frying pan, heat the remaining oil over low heat and sauté the garlic, wax peppers, all kinds of paprika and caraway seeds for about 20-30 seconds.

Remove from the heat and set aside.

In a small bowl, mix together the gelatin and broth.

In the large pan, add the cooked pork, garlic mixture, gelatin mixture and bay leaf and bring t0 a gentle boil.

Reduce the heat to low and simmer, covered for about 2 hours.

Stir in the xanthan gum and simmer for about 3-5 minutes.

Stir in the lemon juice, salt and black pepper and remove from the heat.

Serve hot.

Nutrition:

Calories: 529 Carbohydrates: 5.8g

Protein: 38.9g Fat: 38.5g Sugar: 2.6g

Sodium: 216mg Fiber: 2.1g

Yellow Chicken Soup

Cooking Time: 25 minutes

Preparation Time: 15 minutes

Servings: 5

Ingredients:

2½ tsp. ground turmeric

1½ tsp. ground cumin

1/8 tsp cayenne pepper

2 tbsp. butter, divided

1 small yellow onion, chopped

2 C. cauliflower, chopped

2 C. broccoli, chopped

4 C. homemade chicken broth

1½ C. water

1 tsp. fresh ginger root, grated

1 bay leaf

2 C. Swiss chard stemmed and chopped finely

½ C. unsweetened coconut milk

3 (4-oz.) grass-fed boneless, skinless chicken thighs, cut into bite-size pieces

2 tbsp. fresh lime juice

Directions:

In a small bowl, mix together the turmeric, cumin and cayenne pepper and set aside.

Ina large pan, melt 1 tbsp. of the butter over medium heat and sauté the onion for about 3-4 minutes.

Add the cauliflower, broccoli and half of the spice mixture and cook for another 3-4 minutes.

Add the broth, water, ginger and bay leaf and bring to a boil.

Reduce the heat to low and simmer for about 8-10 minutes.

Stir in the Swiss chard and coconut milk and cook for about 1-2 minutes.

Meanwhile, in a large skillet, melt the remaining butter over medium heat and sear the chicken pieces for about 5 minutes.

Stir in the remaining spice mix and cook for about 5 minutes, stirring frequently.

Transfer the soup into serving bowls and top with the chicken pieces.

Drizzle with lime juice and serve.

Nutrition:

Calories: 258

Carbohydrates: 8.4g Protein: 18.4g

Fat: 16.8g Sugar: 3g Sodium: 753mg

Fiber: 2.9g

Curry Soup

Preparation Time: 25 minutes

Cooking Time: 20 minutes

Servings: 4

Ingredients:

¾ tsp. cumin

¼ c. pumpkin seeds, raw

½ tsp. Garlic powder

½ tsp. Paprika ½ tsp. sea salt

1 c. coconut milk, unsweetened

1 clove garlic, minced

1 med. onion, diced

2 c. carrots, chopped

2 tbsp. curry powder

3 c. cauliflower, riced

3 tbsp. extra virgin olive oil, divided

4 c. kale, chopped

4 c. vegetable broth

Sea salt & pepper to taste

Directions:

Hear a large saute pan over medium heat with 2 tablespoons of olive oil. Once the oil is hot, add the rice cauliflower to the pan along with the curry powder, cumin, salt, paprika, and garlic powder. Stir thoroughly to combine.

While cooking, stir occasionally. Once the cauliflower is warmed through, remove it from the heat.

In a large pot over medium heat, add the remainder of your olive oil. Once it's hot, add the onion and allow it to cook for about four minutes. Add the garlic, then cook for about another two minutes.

To the large pot, add the broth, kale, carrots, and cauliflower. Stir to incorporate thoroughly.

Allow the mixture to come to a boil, drop the heat to low, and allow the soup to simmer for about 15 minutes.

Stir the coconut milk into the mixture along with salt and pepper to taste.

Garnish with pumpkin seeds and serve hot!

Nutrition:

Calories: 274

Carbs: 11 grams

Fat: 19 grams

Protein: 15 grams

Delicious Tomato Basil Soup

Preparation Time: 10 minutes

Cook Time: 40 minutes

Servings: 4

Ingredients:

¼ c. olive oil

½ c. heavy cream

1 lb. tomatoes, fresh

4 c. chicken broth, divided

4 cloves garlic, fresh

Sea salt & pepper to taste

Directions:

Preheat oven to 400° Fahrenheit and line a baking sheet with foil.

Remove the cores from your tomatoes and place them on the baking sheet along with the cloves of garlic.

Drizzle tomatoes and garlic with olive oil, salt, and pepper.

Roast at 400° Fahrenheit for 30 minutes.

Pull the tomatoes out of the oven and place them into a blender, along with the juices that have dripped onto the pan during roasting.

Add two cups of the chicken broth to the blender.

Blend until smooth, then strain the mixture into a large saucepan or a pot.

While the pan is on the stove, whisk the remaining two cups of broth and the cream into the soup.

Simmer for about ten minutes.

Season to taste, then serve hot!

Nutrition:

Calories: 225 Carbohydrates: 5.5 grams

Fat: 20 grams Protein: 6.5 grams

Chicken Enchilada Soup

Preparation Time: 10 minutes

Cooking Time: 45 minutes

Servings: 4

Ingredients:

½ c. fresh cilantro, chopped

1 ¼ tsp. chili powder

1 c. fresh tomatoes, diced

1 med. yellow onion, diced

1 sm. red bell pepper, diced

1 tbsp. cumin, ground

1 tbsp. extra virgin olive oil

1 tbsp. lime juice, fresh

1 tsp. dried oregano

2 cloves garlic, minced

2 lg. stalks celery, diced

4 c. chicken broth

8 oz. chicken thighs, boneless & skinless, shredded

8 oz. cream cheese, softened

Directions:

In a pot over medium heat, warm olive oil.

Once hot, add celery, red pepper, onion, and garlic. Cook for about 3 minutes or until shiny.

Stir the tomatoes into the pot and let cook for another 2 minutes.

Add seasonings to the pot, stir in chicken broth and bring to a boil.

Once boiling, drop the heat down to low and allow to simmer for 20 minutes.

Once simmering, add the cream cheese and allow the soup to return to a boil. *

Drop the heat once again and allow it to simmer for another 20 minutes.

Stir the shredded chicken into the soup along with the lime juice and the cilantro.

Spoon into bowls and serve hot!

Nutrition:

Calories: 420 Carbohydrates: 9 grams

Fat: 29.5 grams Protein: 27 grams

Buffalo Chicken Soup

Preparation Time: 20 minutes

Cook Time: 20 minutes

Servings: 4

Ingredients:

4 med. stalks celery, diced

2 med. carrots, diced

4 chicken breasts, boneless & skinless

6 tbsp. butter - 1 qt. chicken broth

2 oz. cream cheese - ½ c. heavy cream

½ c. buffalo sauce 1 tsp. sea salt

½ tsp. thyme, dried

For garnish:

Sour cream - Green onions, thinly sliced

Bleu cheese crumbles

Directions:

Set a large pot to warm over medium heat with the olive oil in it.

Cook celery and carrot until shiny and tender. Add chicken breasts to the pot and cover. Allow cooking about five to six minutes per side. Once the chicken has cooked and formed some caramelization on each side, remove it from the pot.

Shred the chicken breasts and set aside. Pour the chicken broth into the pot with the carrots and celery, then stir in the cream, butter, and cream cheese. * Bring the pot to a boil, then add the chicken back to the pool. Stir buffalo sauce into the mix and combine thoroughly. Feel free to increase or decrease as desired.

Add seasonings, stir, and drop the heat to low. Allow the soup to simmer for 15 to 20 minutes, or until all the flavors have thoroughly combined. Serve hot with a garnish of sour cream, bleu cheese crumbles, and sliced green onion!

Nutrition:

Calories: 563 Carbohydrates: 4 grams

Fat: 32.5 grams Protein: 57 grams

Slow Cooker Taco Soup

Preparation Time: 10 minutes

Cooking Time: 2 hours

Servings: 8

Ingredients:

¼ c. sour cream

½ c. cheddar cheese, shredded

2 c. diced tomatoes

2 lbs. ground beef

3 tbsp. taco seasoning*

4 c. chicken broth

8 oz. cream cheese, cubed**

Directions:

Heat a medium saucepan over medium heat and brown the beef.

Drain the fat from the beef and then place it into the slow cooker.

Add the cream cheese cubes, taco seasoning, and diced tomatoes into the slow cooker.

Add the chicken broth, cover and leave to cook on high for two hours. Once the timer is up, stir all the ingredients and spoon the soup into bowls.

Serve hot with sour cream and shredded cheese on top!

*Check the label! Make sure that the taco seasoning you buy doesn't contain hidden sugars or starches.

**Cream cheese is more comfortable to cut when it's freezing, and if you carefully spread a little bit of olive oil on the blade of the knife!

Nutrition:

Calories: 505 Carbohydrates: 8.5 grams

Fat: 31.5 grams Protein: 43.5 grams

Wedding Soup

Preparation Time: 5 minutes

Cooking Time: 10 minutes

Servings: 4

Ingredients:

½ c. almond flour

½ c. parmesan cheese, grated

½ sm. yellow onion, diced

1 lb. ground beef

1 lb. egg, beaten

1 tsp. Italian seasoning

1 tsp. oregano, fresh & chopped

1 tsp. thyme, mint & chopped

2 c. baby leaf spinach, fresh

2 c. cauliflower, riced

2 med. stalks celery, diced

2 tbsp. extra virgin olive oil

3 cloves garlic, minced

6 c. chicken broth

Sea salt & pepper to taste

Directions:

In a large mixing bowl, combine almond flour, parmesan cheese, ground beef, egg, salt, pepper, and Italian seasoning. Mix thoroughly by a band

Shape the meat mixture into one-inch meatballs, cover, and refrigerate until ready to cook.

In a large saucepan over medium heat, warm the olive oil. Once the oil is hot, stir the celery and onion into the pan and season to taste with salt and pepper.

Stirring often, bring the onion and celery to a lightly cooked state, about six or seven minutes.

Add the garlic to the pan, stir to combine, and allow to cook for one more minute.

Stir chicken broth, fresh oregano, and the fresh thyme into the pan and stir to combine.

Bring the mixture to a boil.

Drop the heat to low and allow to simmer for about ten minutes before adding cauliflower and meatballs to it. Allow to cool for about five minutes or until the meatballs are cooked all the way through. Add the spinach to the soup and stir in for about one to two minutes, or until it's sufficiently wilted.

Add seasoning as is needed.

Serve hot!

Nutrition:

Calories: 420 Carbohydrates: 4 grams

Fat: 26 grams

Protein: 6.5 grams

CHAPTER 22:

Dessert Recipes

Chocolate Lava Cake

Preparation Time: 3 minutes

Cooking Time: 10 minutes

Servings: 4

Ingredients::

½ cup raw unsweetened cocoa powder

¼ cup butter, melted

4 eggs

¼ cup sugar-free and gluten-free chocolate sauce

½ teaspoon ground cinnamon

½ teaspoon of sea salt

1 teaspoon pure vanilla extract

¼ cup raw stevia

Directions:

Pour 1 tablespoon of chocolate sauce into 4 cavities of an ice cube tray and freeze it.

Preheat oven to 350°F. Prepare 4 ramekins by greasing with oil or butter.

Whisk together the cocoa powder, stevia, cinnamon, and sea salt in a small bowl.

Whisk in the eggs, one at a time.

Add the melted butter and vanilla extract. Stir until well combined.

Fill each prepared ramekin halfway with the mixture.

Remove the chocolate sauce from the freezer and place one in each of the ramekins.

Cover the chocolate with the remaining cake batter.

Bake for 13 to 14 minutes or until just set. Transfer from the oven to a wire rack and allow to cool for 5 minutes.

Carefully remove the cakes from the ramekins.

Enjoy your tasty and healthy chocolate lava cake by cutting into its molten center.

Nutrition:

Total Carbohydrates: 6g

Protein: 8g Dietary Fiber: 3g

Total Fat: 17g Net Carbs: 3g Calories: 189

Decadent Three-Layered Chocolate Cream Cake

Preparation Time: 30 minutes

Cooking Time: 30 minutes

Servings: 8

Ingredients::

4 ounces unsweetened chocolate

½ cup (1 stick) butter

1 ½ cups powdered sweetener, divided

3 eggs

½ cup + 8 tablespoons raw unsweetened cocoa powder

1 vanilla pod

Pinch of sea salt

1 cup whipping cream

Coconut whipped cream

1 can coconut milk, refrigerated overnight

Directions:

Preheat the oven to 325°F. Spray a little cooking oil into a pan smaller than 8 inches.

Combine the chocolate and butter in a double boiler and melt them together. Stir in ½ cup of sweetener and keep on stirring over low heat until everything is well combined. Remove from heat and let cool a little bit.

Separate the eggs, and beat the whites until stiff peaks form. Add ¼ cup of sweetener little by little.

Whisk the yolks together with another ¼ cup of sweetener. Add the chocolate mixture to the yolks and stir well. Mix in ½ cup cocoa, and then scrape the vanilla seeds from the pod and add to the mix along with salt.

Fold in egg whites slowly to the chocolate mixture, but do not over mix.

Cook in the preheated oven for 1 hour or until a toothpick comes out clean. Let it cool completely and then remove from the pan.

Cream:

To prepare the 3 types of filling, beat the whipping cream for about 6-7 minutes until it gets very thick. Slowly add ½ cup of sweetener.

Divide the cream into halves and place one half in a bowl. Divide the remaining cream into halves again and place it in the other 2 separate bowls. You will have 3 bowls, one with ½ of the cream and two with ¼ of the cream.

Take a bowl with ¼ cream, add 1 tablespoon of cocoa powder and mix well. This will be the lightest-colored cream.

Add ½ the cream to the bowl, add 3 tablespoons of cocoa powder. Mix until well distributed. This will be the middle-colored cream. Add 3–4 tablespoons of cocoa powder to the last bowl with ¼ cream. This will be the darkest cream.

Assembling:

Slice the cake horizontally in 3 equal slices using a very sharp knife. Place the bottom part on a serving plate and cover with the middle-colored cream. Repeat with the second layer. Top with the third cake piece and spread the light-colored cream on top, followed by the darkest cream. Cut in 8 slices and enjoy.

Nutrition:

Total Carbohydrates: 11g Protein: 7g

Dietary Fiber: 6g Total Fat: 27g

Net Carbs: 5g Calories: 304

Individual Strawberry Cheesecakes

Preparation Time: 10 minutes

Cooking Time: 0 minute

Servings: 4

Ingredients::

Crust

½ cup almond flour

3 tablespoons butter, melted (use coconut oil for a paleo version)

¼ cup sugar substitute (use pure Grade B maple syrup for a paleo version)

Filling

6 strawberries

3 tablespoons sugar substitute (use pure Grade B maple syrup for a paleo version)

8 ounces cream cheese (use full-fat unsweetened coconut cream for a paleo version)

1/3 cup sour cream (eliminate for a paleo version)

½ teaspoon pure vanilla extract

4 strawberries, quartered (for garnish)

Fresh mint leaves (optional for garnish)

Directions:

To prepare the crust, place the almond flour, melted butter, and sugar substitute in a medium bowl and mix well to combine.

Divide the mixture evenly into 4 small serving bowls or ramekins, lightly pressing with your hands.

To prepare the filling, puree the strawberries in a food processor.

Add the sugar substitute, vanilla extract, cream cheese, and sour cream. Blend until smooth and creamy.

Spoon the mixture over the crust and chill for at least 1 hour.

Nutrition:

Total Carbohydrates: 12g

Protein: 8g Dietary Fiber: 3g

Total Fat: 47g Net Carbs: 9g Calories: 489

Brownie Cheesecake Bars

Preparation Time: 5 minutes

Cooking Time: 50 minutes

Servings: 6

Ingredients::

Brownie layer:

2 ounces bittersweet chocolate, chopped

½ cup butter softened

⅓ cup raw unsweetened cocoa powder

½ cup almond flour

2 large eggs - ½ cup sugar substitute

½ teaspoon pure vanilla extract

¼ teaspoon salt - Cheesecake layer

2 large eggs - 16 ounces cream cheese, softened

⅓ cup sugar substitute - ¼ cup heavy cream

½ teaspoon pure vanilla extract

Directions:

Preheat oven to 325°F.

Grease an 8x8 glass baking dish with butter or oil.

Melt the chocolate and butter together in a small saucepan over medium heat. Stir until well combined.

Whisk the almond flour, cocoa powder, and salt together in a small bowl.

Whisk the eggs, sugar substitute, and vanilla extract in a large bowl until frothy. Slowly whisk in the melted chocolate mixture.

Stir in the almond flour mixture and mix until smooth.

Pour into the prepared baking dish and bake for 20 minutes. Transfer to a wire rack and allow to cool.

For the cheesecake layer, mix together the cream cheese, eggs, sugar substitute, heavy cream, and vanilla extract with an electric mixer.

Reduce the oven heat to 300°F. Pour the batter over the baked brownies and return to the oven for 40 to 45 minutes or until set.

Remove from the oven and cool in the fridge for at least 2 hours prior to serving.

Nutrition:

Total Carbohydrates: 12g Protein: 13g

Dietary Fiber: 3g Total Fat: 54g

Net Carbs: 9g Calories: 566

Rich Chocolate Pudding

Preparation Time: 5 minutes

Cooking Time: 5 minutes

Servings: 4

Ingredients::

2 cups coconut milk, canned

¼ cup raw unsweetened cocoa powder

1 tablespoon stevia

2 tablespoons gelatin

4 tablespoons water

½ cup heavy whipping cream, beaten to stiff peaks

1 ounce chopped bittersweet chocolate (optional for garnish)

Directions:

Heat the coconut milk, cocoa powder, and stevia in a small saucepan over medium heat. Stir until the cocoa powder and stevia have dissolved.

Mix the gelatin with the water and add to the saucepan. Stir until well combined.

Pour the mixture into 4 small ramekins or glasses.

Place the ramekins in the refrigerator for at least 1 hour.

Top with whipped cream, and chopped chocolate, if desired.

Nutrition:

Total Carbohydrates: 14g

Protein: 8g

Dietary Fiber: 5g

Total Fat: 37g

Net Carbs: 10g

Calories: 389

Fresh Strawberries with Coconut Whip

Preparation Time: 5 minutes

Cooking Time: 3 minutes

Servings: 4

Ingredients::

2 cans coconut cream, refrigerated

4 cups strawberries (can also use blueberries, blackberries, raspberries, or a combination)

1 ounce chopped unsweetened 70% or darker dark chocolate

Directions:

Scoop the solidified coconut cream (reserving the liquid in the bottom of the can for another use) into a large bowl and blend with a hand mixer on high for about 5 minutes or until stiff peaks form.

Slice the strawberries and arrange them in 4 small serving bowls.

Dollop the coconut whipped cream on top of the strawberries.

Garnish with chopped dark chocolate and additional berries.

Serve and enjoy!

Nutrition:

Total Carbohydrates: 15g

Protein: 4g

Dietary Fiber: 5g

Total Fat: 31g

Net Carbs: 10g

Calories: 342

Choco-Nut Milkshake

Preparation Time: 5 minutes

Cooking Time: 0 minute

Servings: 4

Ingredients:

2 cups unsweetened coconut, almond, or dairy-free milk of choice

1 banana, sliced and frozen

¼ cup unsweetened coconut flakes

1 cup of ice cubes

¼ cup macadamia nuts, chopped

3 tablespoons sugar-free sweetener (use pure Grade B maple syrup for a paleo version)

2 tablespoons raw unsweetened cocoa powder

Whipped coconut cream (optional for garnish)

Directions:

Place all **Ingredients:** into a blender and blend on high until smooth and creamy.

Divide evenly between 4 "mocktail" glasses and top with whipped coconut cream, if desired.

Add a cocktail umbrella and toasted coconut for added flair.

Enjoy your delicious choco-nut smoothie!

Nutrition:

Total Carbohydrates: 12g

Protein: 3g

Dietary Fiber: 4g

Total Fat: 17g

Net Carbs: 8g

Calories: 199

Butter Pecan Ice Cream

Preparation Time: 10 minutes

Cooking Time: 0 minute

Servings: 4

Ingredients:

½ cup chopped pecans

1/8 teaspoon xanthan gum

2 egg yolks

1 teaspoon pure vanilla extract

¼ cup sugar substitute

2 tablespoons butter

1 cup heavy cream

Directions:

Melt the butter in a small saucepan over medium heat. Whisk the heavy cream into the butter after it has melted and become slightly brown.

Stir in the sugar substitute and mix until dissolved.

Add the xanthan gum and whisk until well combined. Transfer to a large, metal bowl and allow it to cool.

Add the egg yolks slowly, one at a time, using a hand mixer.

Stir in the pecans and vanilla extract.

Place the bowl in the freezer for at least 4 hours, stirring well every hour.

Remove from the freezer and scoop into serving bowls.

Garnish with additional chopped pecans, if desired, and serve!

Nutrition:

Total Carbohydrates: 2g Protein: 3g

Dietary Fiber: 1g Total Fat: 24g

Net Carbs: 1g Calories: 230

No-Churn Blueberry Ice Cream

Preparation Time: 15 minutes

Cooking Time: 0 minute

Servings: 4

Ingredients:

¼ cup crème fraîche or sour cream (be sure to check the label for GF labeling)

1 cup heavy whipping cream

¼ cup fresh blueberries

1 egg yolk, beaten

2 teaspoons pure vanilla extract

Directions:

Whip the crème fraîche with a hand mixer until frothy.

Whip the heavy cream in a separate bowl until soft peaks form.

Fold the crème fraîche into the whipped cream carefully.

Puree the blueberries in a food processor or blender until smooth.

Stir the blueberry puree, egg yolk, and vanilla extract into the whipped cream mixture. Mix until just combined.

Transfer mixture into a loaf pan and freeze for 2 hours, stirring well every 30 minutes.

Scoop into serving bowls and enjoy your fresh blueberry ice cream!

Nutrition:

Total Carbohydrates: 3g

Protein: 2g Dietary Fiber: 0g

Total Fat: 15g Net Carbs: 3g

Calories: 153

Carrot Cake with Cream Cheese Frosting

Preparation Time: 15 minutes

Cooking Time: 30 minutes

Servings: 6

Ingredients:

Carrot cake

1½ cups carrots, grated finely

¾ cups sugar substitute

¼ cup brown sugar substitute

½ cup coconut oil, melted

2 large eggs

¼ cup flax meal

½ teaspoon baking soda

½ teaspoon ground cinnamon

¼ teaspoon ground nutmeg

¾ cup almond flour

Cream Cheese Frosting

8 ounces cream cheese, softened

2 tablespoons pure Grade B maple syrup

¼ teaspoon pure vanilla extract

¼ cup toasted walnuts, chopped (optional for garnish)

Directions:

Preheat oven to 350°F. Grease a 9-inch round cake pan with butter or oil.

Blend the sugars, coconut oil, and eggs using a hand mixer.

Whisk the dry ingredients together in a separate bowl until well combined.

Add the dry ingredients slowly and keep blending until no lumps remain.

Stir in the grated carrots and pour into the prepared cake pan. Bake for 30 minutes or until a toothpick inserted comes out clean.

Remove from oven and allow cooling

To prepare the frosting, beat the cream cheese, maple syrup, and vanilla extract until light and fluffy.

Top the cake with the frosting, sprinkle with toasted walnuts, slice and serve!

Nutrition:

Total Carbohydrates: 14g

Protein: 11g

Dietary Fiber: 5g

Total Fat: 45g

Net Carbs: 9g

Calories: 479

Peanut Butter Cookies

Preparation Time: 5 Minutes

Cooking Time: 15 Minutes

Servings: 4

Ingredients:

½ cup peanut butter

½ cup powdered erythritol

1 egg

Directions:

Preheat your oven to 350 degrees F.

Layer a baking sheet with wax paper and set it aside.

Add all the ingredients to a bowl and mix well to prepare the cookie dough.

Add 1.5 tablespoons of the dough on the baking sheet scoop by scoop to make the cookies.

Bake for 15 minutes until golden brown.

Enjoy.

Nutrition:

Calories 179

Total Fat 15.7 g

Saturated Fat 8 g

Cholesterol 323mg

Sodium 43 mg

Total Carbs 4.8 g

Sugar 3.6 g

Fiber 0.8 g

Protein 5.6 g

Mint Creme Oreos

Preparation Time: 10 Minutes

Cooking Time: 12 Minutes

Servings: 12

Ingredients:

2 ¼ cups almond flour

3 tbsp coconut flour

4 tbsp cacao powder

1 tsp baking powder

1 ½ tsp xanthan gum

¼ tsp salt

½ cup grass-fed butter, unsalted and softened

1 egg

1 tsp vanilla extract

4 oz cream cheese

1 cup lakanto monk fruit

1 tsp peppermint extract

Directions:

Preheat your oven to 350 degrees F.

Mix coconut flour with almond flour, xanthan gum, salt, baking powder, and cocoa powder in a medium-sized bowl.

Whisk ½ cup monk fruit sweetener with six tablespoons of butter in a bowl until fluffy.

Add vanilla extract and egg, then beat well and stir in dry ingredients to form the dough.

Place this dough in between two sheets of wax paper and roll it into a 1/8-inch thick sheet.

Cut cookies with a round cookie cutter then re-roll the remaining dough to cut more cookies.

Place these cookies on a cookie sheet lined with parchment paper.

Bake these cookies for 12 minutes then allow them to cool.

Meanwhile, beat cream cheese with 2 tablespoons butter, ½ cup monk fruit, and peppermint extract in a small bowl.

Divide this mixture over half of the cookies.

Place the remaining half of the cookies over the cream filling

Press the two halves together gently.

Enjoy.

Nutrition:

Calories 331 Total Fat 12.9 g

Saturated Fat 6.1 g   Cholesterol 10 mg

Sodium 18 mg

Total Carbs 9.1 g

Sugar 2.8 g

Fiber 0.8 g

Protein 4.4 g

Butter Glazed Cookies

Preparation Time: 15 Minutes

Cooking Time: 6 Minutes

Servings: 40 Cookies

Ingredients:

1/3 cup coconut flour - 2/3 cup almond flour

¼ cup granulated erythritol - 8 drops stevia

½ cup butter softened

1 tsp almond or vanilla extract

¼ tsp baking powder

¼ tsp xanthan gum (optional)

For the Glaze:

¼ cup coconut butter - 8 drops stevia

Directions:

Preheat your oven to 356 degrees F. Whisk dry ingredients in one bowl and beat butter with stevia and vanilla extract in another. Add dry mixture and mix well until smooth, then divide the dough into two pieces. Place each dough piece in between two sheets of wax paper. Spread them into a thick sheet and refrigerate for 10 minutes. Use a cookies cutter to cut small cookies out of both the dough sheets. Place them on a baking sheet lined with wax paper and bake them for 6 minutes. Meanwhile, prepare the glaze by heating coconut butter with stevia in a bowl in the microwave. Pour this glaze over each cookie and allow it to set. Serve.

Nutrition:

Calories 237 Total Fat 22 g

Saturated Fat 9 g Cholesterol 35 mg

Sodium 118 mg Total Carbs 5 g Sugar 1 g

Fiber 2 g Protein 5 g

Pecan Shortbread Cookies

Preparation Time: 5 Minutes

Cooking Time: 15 Minutes

Servings: 6

Ingredients:

¾ cup almond flour

¼ cup coconut flour

1 large egg

4 tbsp butter, melted

½ cup erythritol

1 tsp vanilla extract

½ tsp baking powder

¼ tsp xanthan gum

1/3 cup raw pecans, crushed

Directions:

Add all dry Ingredient to a bowl then mix well with a fork.

Whisk melted butter and vanilla extract in a separate bowl, then stir in half of the dry mixture.

Add egg and mix well until combined. Now, stir in the remaining dry mixture.

Mix this well until fully incorporated.

Add pecans to the cookie dough and mix well.

Place the dough on wax paper and form it into a rectangular log with your hands.

Cover it with more wax paper and freeze for 30 minutes.

Meanwhile, preheat your oven for 5 minutes at 350 degrees F.

Layer a cookie sheet with wax paper and set it aside.

Slice the dough log into ¼-inch thick slices.

Place the slices on the cookie sheet and bake them for 15 minutes.

Allow them to cool then serve.

Nutrition:

Calories 121

Total Fat 12.9 g

Saturated Fat 5.1 g

Cholesterol 17 mg

Sodium 28 mg

Total Carbs 8.1 g

Sugar 1.8 g

Fiber 0.4 g

Protein 5.4 g

Pistachio Cookies

Preparation Time: 10 Minutes

Cooking Time: 25 Minutes

Servings: 8

Ingredients:

¾ cup (4 oz) shelled pistachio nuts

2 tsp + 1 cup stevia granulated sweetener

1 2/3 cup almond meal or almond flour

2 eggs, beaten well

Directions:

Add pistachio and stevia to a food processor and pulse until finely ground.

Toss pistachio mixture with almond meal or flour in a bowl.

Add eggs and whisk well until combined.

Refrigerate this mixture for 8 hours or overnight.

Let your oven preheat at 325 degrees F.

Layer a cookie sheet with wax paper then use a scoop or spoon to add the cookie dough to the sheet scoop by scoop.

Bake them for 25 minutes until lightly brown.

Allow them to cool then serve.

Nutrition:

Calories 174

Total Fat 12.3 g

Saturated Fat 4.8 g

Cholesterol 32 mg

Sodium 597 mg

Total Carbs 4.5 g

Fiber 0.6 g

Sugar 1.9 g

Protein 12 g

Chocolate Dipped Cookies

Preparation Time: 10 Minutes

Cooking Time: 30 Minutes

Servings: 8

Ingredients:

1 ½ cups almond flour

¼ cup almond butter

2 tbsp powdered erythritol

1 large egg

1 tsp vanilla powder

1 tbsp virgin coconut oil

1 tbsp coconut butter

1 tsp baking powder

Pinch of salt

3.2 oz 90% dark chocolate

Directions:

Whisk almond flour, vanilla, salt, baking powder, and erythritol in a mixing bowl.

Stir in almond butter, egg, coconut butter, and coconut oil.

Mix well to form a dough then place it in a sandwich bag. Refrigerate for 30 minutes.

Let your oven preheat at 285 degrees F.

Place the dough in between two sheets of parchment then roll it into a ½-inch thick sheet.

Use a 2.5-inch diameter cookie cutter to cut the cookies out of this dough.

Reroll the remaining dough then place it on a greased baking sheet.

Bake the cookies for 30 minutes until golden brown.

Place them on a wire rack to cool down.

Melt chocolate in a bowl by heating in a microwave and stir well.

Dip half of each cooled cookie in the chocolate melt and allow it to set on wax paper.

Refrigerate the dipped cookies for 15 minutes.

Serve.

Nutrition:

Calories 236

Total Fat 13.5 g Saturated Fat 4.2 g

Cholesterol 541 mg Sodium 21 mg

Total Carbs 7.6 g Sugar 1.4 g

Fiber 3.8 g Protein 4.3 g

Shortbread Cookies

Preparation Time: 10 Minutes

Cooking Time: 13 Minutes

Servings: 6

Ingredients:

1 ½ cups almond flour

½ tsp xanthan gum

¼ tsp kosher salt

6 tbsp grass-fed butter, room temperature

6 tbsp powdered erythritol

½ tsp vanilla extract

Directions:

Spread almond flour in a dry skillet and place it over medium heat.

Stir cook for 3 minutes or more until golden brown then removes it from the heat.

Add salt and xanthan gum to the flour and mix well.

Beat butter with an electric mixer for 3 minutes and add sweetener.

Continue beating, then add vanilla extract. Beat until combined.

Add almond flour mixture and whisk well until it forms a smooth dough.

Wrap the dough in a plastic wrap then refrigerate for 1 hour.

Let your oven preheat at 350 degrees F and grease a baking tray with cooking oil.

Place the cookie dough between two parchment sheets and roll it into a ¼-inch thick sheet.

Cut out cookies using any shape cookie cutter.

Arrange all the cookies on a baking sheet and freeze for 15 minutes.

Bake them for 13 minutes until golden brown.

Serve.

Nutrition:

Calories 167 Total Fat 5.1 g

Saturated Fat 1.1 g Cholesterol 121 mg

Sodium 48 mg Total Carbs 8.9 g

Sugar 3.8 g Fiber 2.1 g Protein 6.3 g

Stuffed Oreo Cookies

Preparation Time: 10 Minutes

Cooking Time: 12 Minutes

Servings: 12

Ingredients:

1 1/3 cup almond flour

6 tbsp cocoa powder

2 tbsp black cocoa powder

¾ tsp kosher salt

½ tsp xanthan gum

½ tsp baking soda

¼ tsp espresso powder

5 ½ tbsp butter

8 tbsp erythritol

1 egg

For Vanilla Cream Filling

4 tbsp grass-fed butter

1 tbsp coconut oil

1 ½ tsp vanilla extract

Pinch kosher salt

½ - 1 cup Swerve confectioner sugar substitute

Directions:

Whisk almond flour, salt, both cocoa powders, xanthan gum, baking soda, and espresso powder in a suitable bowl.

Beat butter well in a large bowl with a hand mixer for 2 minutes.

Whisk in sweetener and continue beating for 5 minutes, then add the egg.

Beat well, then add the flour mixture. Mix well until fully incorporated.

Wrap the cookie dough with plastic wrap and refrigerate for 1 hour.

Meanwhile, preheat your oven to 350 degrees F and layer a baking sheet with wax paper.

Place the dough in between two sheets of parchment paper.

Roll the dough out into a 1/8-inch thick sheet.

Cut 1 ¾ inch round cookies out of this sheet and reroll the dough to cut more cookies.

Spread these cookies on the baking sheet and freeze for 15 minutes.

Bake these cookies for 12 minutes then allow them to cool on a wire rack.

Beat butter with coconut oil in a bowl with an electric mixer.

Stir in vanilla extract, powdered sweetener to taste, and a pinch of salt.

Mix well then transfer it to a piping bag.

Place half of the cookies on a cookie sheet and top them with the cream filling.

Place the remaining half of the cookies over the filling to cover it

Refrigerate for 15 minutes then serve.

Nutrition:

Calories 356

Total Fat 7.1 g

Saturated Fat 2.1 g

Cholesterol 113 mg

Sodium 72 mg

Total Carbs 3.9 g

Sugar 3.7 g

Fiber 2.3 g

Protein 6.3 g

CHAPTER 23:

Snacks Recipes

Fluffy Bites

Preparation Time: 20 minutes

Cooking Time: 60 minutes

Servings: 12

Ingredients:

2 Teaspoons Cinnamon

2/3 Cup Sour Cream

2 Cups Heavy Cream

1 Teaspoon Scraped Vanilla Bean

¼ Teaspoon Cardamom

4 Egg Yolks

Stevia to Taste

Directions:

Start by whisking your egg yolks until creamy and smooth.

Get out a double boiler, and add your eggs with the rest of your ingredients. Mix well.

Remove from heat, allowing it to cool until it reaches room temperature.

Refrigerate for an hour before whisking well.

Pour into molds, and freeze for at least an hour before serving.

Nutrition:

Calories: 363 Protein: 2

Fat: 40 Carbohydrates: 1

Coconut Fudge

Preparation Time: 20 minutes

Cooking Time: 60 minutes

Servings: 12

Ingredients:

2 Cups Coconut Oil

½ Cup Dark Cocoa Powder

½ Cup Coconut Cream

¼ Cup Almonds, Chopped

¼ Cup Coconut, Shredded

1 Teaspoon Almond Extract

Pinch of Salt

Stevia to Taste

Directions:

Pour your coconut oil and coconut cream in a bowl, whisking with an electric beater until smooth. Once the mixture becomes smooth and glossy, do not continue.

Begin to add in your cocoa powder while mixing slowly, making sure that there aren't any lumps.

Add in the rest of your ingredients, and mix well.

Line a bread pan with parchment paper, and freeze until it sets.

Slice into squares before serving.

Nutrition:

Calories: 172 Fat: 20 Carbohydrates: 3

Nutmeg Nougat

Preparation Time: 30 minutes

Cooking Time: 60 minutes

Servings: 12

Ingredients:

1 Cup Heavy Cream - 1 Cup Cashew Butter

1 Cup Coconut, Shredded - ½ Teaspoon Nutmeg

1 Teaspoon Vanilla Extract, Pure

Stevia to Taste

Directions:

Melt your cashew butter using a double boiler, and then stir in your vanilla extract, dairy cream, nutmeg and stevia. Make sure it's mixed well.

Remove from heat, allowing it to cool down before refrigerating it for a half-hour.

Shape into balls, and coat with shredded coconut. Chill for at least two hours before serving.

Nutrition:

Calories: 341 Fat: 34 arbohydrates: 5

Sweet Almond Bites

Preparation Time: 30 minutes

Cooking Time: 90 minutes

Servings: 12

Ingredients:

18 Ounces Butter, Grass-Fed

2 Ounces Heavy Cream

½ Cup Stevia

2/3 Cup Cocoa Powder

1 Teaspoon Vanilla Extract, Pure

4 Tablespoons Almond Butter

Directions:

Use a double boiler to melt your butter before adding in all of your remaining ingredients.

Place the mixture into molds, freezing for two hours before serving.

Nutrition:

Calories: 350

Protein: 2

Fat: 38

Strawberry Cheesecake Minis

Preparation Time: 30 minutes

Cooking Time: 120 minutes

Servings: 12

Ingredients:

1 Cup Coconut Oil

1 Cup Coconut Butter

½ Cup Strawberries, Sliced

½ Teaspoon Lime Juice

2 Tablespoons Cream Cheese, Full Fat

Stevia to Taste

Directions:

Blend your strawberries together.

Soften your cream cheese, and then add in your coconut butter.

Combine all ingredients, and then pour your mixture into silicone molds.

Freeze for at least two hours before serving.

Nutrition:

Calories: 372 Protein: 1 Fat: 41

Carbohydrates: 2

Cocoa Brownies

Preparation Time: 10 minutes

Cooking Time: 30 minutes

Servings: 12

Ingredients:

1 Egg

2 Tablespoons Butter, Grass Fed

2 Teaspoons Vanilla Extract, Pure

¼ Teaspoon Baking Powder

¼ Cup Cocoa Powder

1/3 Cup Heavy Cream

¾ Cup Almond Butter

Pinch Sea Salt

Directions:

Break your egg into a bowl, whisking until smooth.

Add in all of your wet ingredients, mixing well.

Mix all dry ingredients into a bowl.

Sift your dry ingredients into your wet ingredients, mixing to form a batter.

Get out a baking pan, greasing it before pouring in your mixture.

Heat your oven to 350 and bake for twenty-five minutes.

Allow it to cool before slicing and serve room temperature or warm.

Nutrition:

Calories: 184

Protein: 1

Fat: 20

Carbohydrates: 1

Chocolate Orange Bites

Preparation Time:20 minutes

Cooking Time: 120 minutes

Servings: 6

Ingredients:

10 Ounces Coconut Oil

4 Tablespoons Cocoa Powder

¼ Teaspoon Blood Orange Extract

Stevia to Taste

Directions:

Melt half of your coconut oil using a double boiler, and then add in your stevia and orange extract.

Get out candy molds, pouring the mixture into it. Fill each mold halfway, and then place in the fridge until they set.

Melt the other half of your coconut oil, stirring in your cocoa powder and stevia, making sure that the mixture is smooth with no lumps.

Pour into your molds, filling them up all the way, and then allow it to set in the fridge before serving.

Nutrition:

Calories: *188*

Protein: *1*

Fat: 21

Carbohydrates: 5

Caramel Cones

Preparation Time: 25 minutes

Cooking Time: 120 minutes

Servings: 6

Ingredients:

2 Tablespoons Heavy Whipping Cream

2 Tablespoons Sour Cream

1 Tablespoon Caramel Sugar

1 Teaspoon Sea Salt, Fine

1/3 Cup Butter, Grass-Fed

1/3 Cup Coconut Oil

Stevia to Taste

Directions:

Soften your coconut oil and butter, mixing.

Mix all ingredients to form a batter, and then place them in molds.

Top with a little salt, and keep refrigerated until serving.

Nutrition:

Calories: *100* Fat: 12 Grams Carbohydrates: 1

Cinnamon Bites

Preparation Time: 20 minutes

Cooking Time: 95 minutes

Servings: 6

Ingredients:

1/8 Teaspoon Nutmeg

1 Teaspoon Vanilla Extract

¼ Teaspoon Cinnamon

4 Tablespoons Coconut Oil

½ Cup Butter, Grass-Fed

8 Ounces Cream Cheese

Stevia to Taste

Directions:

Soften your coconut oil and butter, mixing in your cream cheese.

Add all of your remaining ingredients, and mix well.

Pour into molds, and freeze until set.

Nutrition:

Calories: *178* Protein: *1* Fat: 19

Sweet Chai Bites

Preparation Time: 20 minutes

Cooking Time: 45 minutes

Servings: 6

Ingredients:

1 Cup Cream Cheese

1 Cup Coconut Oil

2 Ounces Butter, Grass-Fed

2 Teaspoons Ginger

2 Teaspoons Cardamom

1 Teaspoon Nutmeg

1 Teaspoon Cloves

1 Teaspoon Vanilla Extract, Pure

1 Teaspoon Darjeeling Black Tea

Stevia to Taste

Directions:

Melt your coconut oil and butter before adding in your black tea. Allow it to set for one to two minutes.

Add in your cream cheese, removing your mixture from heat.

Add in all of your spices, and stir to combine.

Pour into molds, and freeze before serving.

Nutrition:

Calories: *178* Protein: *1 Fat:* 19

Easy Vanilla Bombs

Preparation Time: 20 minutes

Cooking Time: 45 minutes

Servings: 14

Ingredients:

1 Cup Macadamia Nuts, Unsalted

¼ Cup Coconut Oil / ¼ Cup Butter

2 Teaspoons Vanilla Extract, Sugar-Free

20 Drops Liquid Stevia

2 Tablespoons Erythritol, Powdered

Directions:

Pulse your macadamia nuts in a blender, and then combine all of your ingredients. Mix well.

Get out mini muffin tins with a tablespoon and a half of the mixture.

Refrigerate it for a half-hour before serving.

Nutrition:

Calories:125

Fat: 5

Carbohydrates: 5

Marinated Eggs.

Preparation Time: 2 hours and 10 minutes

Cooking Time: 7 minutes

Servings: 4

Ingredients:

6 eggs

1 and ¼ cups of water

¼ cup unsweetened rice vinegar 2 tablespoons coconut aminos

Salt and black pepper to the taste 2 garlic cloves, minced

1 teaspoon stevia 4 ounces cream cheese

1 tablespoon chives, chopped

Directions:

Put the eggs in a pot, add water to cover, bring to a boil over medium heat, cover and cook for 7 minutes.

Rinse eggs with cold water and leave them aside to cool down. In a bowl, mix 1 cup water with coconut aminos, vinegar, stevia and garlic and whisk well.

Put the eggs in this mix, cover with a kitchen towel and leave them aside for 2 hours, rotating from time to time.

Peel eggs, cut in halves and put egg yolks in a bowl.

Add ¼ cup water, cream cheese, salt, pepper and chives and stir well.

Stuff egg whites with this mix and serve them.

Enjoy!

Nutrition:

Calories: 289 kcal Protein: 15.86 g

Fat: 22.62 g Carbohydrates: 4.52 g

Sodium: 288 mg

Sausage and Cheese Dip.

Preparation Time: 10 minutes

Cooking Time: 130 minutes

Servings: 28

Ingredients:

8 ounces cream cheese

A pinch of salt and black pepper

16 ounces sour cream

8 ounces pepper jack cheese, chopped

15 ounces canned tomatoes mixed with habaneros

1 pound Italian sausage, ground

¼ cup green onions, chopped

Directions:

Heat a pan over medium heat, add sausage, stir and cook until it browns.

Add tomatoes mix, stir and cook for 4 minutes more.

Add a pinch of salt, pepper and the green onions, stir and cook for 4 minutes.

Spread pepper jack cheese on the bottom of your slow cooker.

Add cream cheese, sausage mix and sour cream, cover and cook on High for 2 hours.

Uncover your slow cooker, stir dip, transfer to a bowl and serve.

Enjoy!

Nutrition:

Calories: 132 kcal

Protein: 6.79 g Fat: 9.58 g

Carbohydrates: 6.22 g

Sodium: 362 mg

Tasty Onion and Cauliflower Dip.

Preparation Time: 20 minutes

Cooking Time: 30 minutes

Servings: 24

Ingredients:

1 and ½ cups chicken stock

1 cauliflower head, florets separated

¼ cup mayonnaise

½ cup yellow onion, chopped

¾ cup cream cheese

½ teaspoon chili powder

½ teaspoon cumin, ground

½ teaspoon garlic powder

Salt and black pepper to the taste

Directions:

Put the stock in a pot, add cauliflower and onion, heat up over medium heat and cook for 30 minutes.

Add chili powder, salt, pepper, cumin and garlic powder and stir.

Also, add cream cheese and stir a bit until it melts.

Blend using an immersion blender and mix with the mayo.

Transfer to a bowl and keep in the fridge for 2 hours before you serve it.

Enjoy!

Nutrition:

Calories: 40 kcal Protein: 1.23 g

Fat: 3.31 g Carbohydrates: 1.66 g

Sodium: 72 mg

Pesto Crackers.

Preparation Time: 10 minutes

Cooking Time: 17 minutes

Servings: 6

Ingredients: ½ teaspoon baking powder

Salt and black pepper to the taste

1 and ¼ cups almond flour ¼ teaspoon basil, dried 1 garlic clove, minced

2 tablespoons basil pesto

A pinch of cayenne pepper

3 tablespoons ghee

Directions:

In a bowl, mix salt, pepper, baking powder and almond flour.

Add garlic, cayenne and basil and stir.

Add pesto and whisk.

Also, add ghee and mix your dough with your finger.

Spread this dough on a lined baking sheet, introduce in the oven at 325 degrees F and bake for 17 minutes.

Leave aside to cool down, cut your crackers and serve them as a snack.

Enjoy!

Nutrition:

Calories: 9 kcal

Protein: 0.41 g

Fat: 0.14 g

Carbohydrates: 1.86 g

Sodium: 2 mg

Pumpkin Muffins.

Preparation Time: 10 minutes

Cooking Time: 15 minutes

Servings: 18

Ingredients:

¼ cup sunflower seed butter

¾ cup pumpkin puree 2 tablespoons flaxseed meal ¼ cup coconut flour

½ cup erythritol ½ teaspoon nutmeg, ground

1 teaspoon cinnamon, ground ½ teaspoon baking soda 1 egg ½ teaspoon baking powder

A pinch of salt

Directions:

In a bowl, mix butter with pumpkin puree and egg and blend well.

Add flaxseed meal, coconut flour, erythritol, baking soda, baking powder, nutmeg, cinnamon and a pinch of salt and stir well.

Spoon this into a greased muffin pan, introduce in the oven at 350 degrees F and bake for 15 minutes.

Leave muffins to cool down and serve them as a snack.

Enjoy!

Nutrition:

Calories: 65 kcal

Protein: 2.82 g

Fat: 5.42 g

Carbohydrates: 2.27 g

Sodium: 57 mg

Creamy Mango and Mint Dip

Preparation Time: 10 minutes

Cooking Time: 15 minutes

Servings: 4

Ingredients:

Medium green chili, chopped – 1

Medium white onion, peeled and chopped – 1

Grated ginger – 1 tablespoon

Minced garlic – 1 teaspoon

Salt – 1/8 teaspoon

Ground black pepper – 1/8 teaspoon

Cumin powder – 1 teaspoon

Mango powder – 1 teaspoon

Mint leaves – 2 cups

Coriander leaves – 1 cup

Cashew yogurt – 4 tablespoons

Directions:

Place all the ingredients for the dip in a blender and pulse for 1 to 2 minutes or until smooth.

Tip the dip into small cups and serve straightaway.

Nutrition:

Calories: 100,

Fat: 2,

Fiber: 3,

Carbs: 7,

Protein: 5

Hot Red Chili and Garlic Chutney

Preparation Time: 25 minutes

Cooking Time: 15 minutes

Servings: 1

Ingredients:

Red chilies, dried – 14

Minced garlic – 5 teaspoons

Salt – 1/8 teaspoon

Water – 1 and ¼ cups

Directions:

Place chilies in a bowl, pour in water and let rest for 20 minutes.

Then drain red chilies, chop them and add to a blender.

Add remaining Ingredients into the blender and pulse for 1 to 2 minutes until smooth.

Tip the sauce into a bowl and serve straight away.

Nutrition:

Calories: 100,

Fat: 1,

Fiber: 2,

Carbs: 6,

Protein: 7

Red Chilies and Onion Chutney

Preparation Time: 15 minutes

Cooking Time: 15 minutes

Servings: 2

Ingredients:

Medium white onion, peeled and chopped – 1

Minced garlic – 1 teaspoon

Red chilies, chopped – 2

Salt – ¼ teaspoon

Sweet paprika – 1 teaspoon

Avocado oil – 2 teaspoons

Water – ¼ cup

Directions:

Place a medium skillet pan over medium-high heat, add oil and when hot, add onion, garlic, and chilies.

Cook onions for 5 minutes or until softened, then season with salt and paprika and pour in water.

Stir well and cook for 5 minutes.

Then spoon the chutney into a bowl and serve.

Nutrition:

Calories: 121,

Fat: 2,

Fiber: 6,

Carbs: 9,

Protein: 5

Fast Guacamole

Preparation Time: 10 minutes

Cooking Time: 15 minutes

Servings: 12

Ingredients:

Medium avocados, peeled, pitted and cubed – 3

Medium tomato, cubed – 1

Chopped cilantro – ¼ cup

Medium red onion, peeled and chopped – 1

Salt – ½ teaspoon

Ground white pepper – ¼ teaspoon

Lime juice – 3 tablespoons

Directions:

Place all the ingredients for the salad in a medium bowl and stir until combined.

Serve guacamole straightaway as an appetizer.

Nutrition:

Calories: 87,

Fat: 4,

Fiber: 4,

Carbs: 8,

Protein: 2

Coconut Dill Dip

Preparation Time: 10 minutes

Cooking Time: 15 minutes

Servings: 10

Ingredients:

Chopped white onion – 1 tablespoon

Parsley flakes – 2 teaspoons

Chopped dill – 2 teaspoons

Salt – ¼ teaspoon

Coconut cream – 1 cup

Avocado mayonnaise – ½ cup

Directions:

Place all the ingredients for the dip in a medium bowl and whisk until combined.

Serve the dip with vegetable sticks as a side dish.

Nutrition:

Calories: 102, Fat: 3, Fiber: 1, Carbs: 2, Protein: 2

Creamy Crab Dip

Preparation Time 5 minutes

Cooking Time: 10 minutes

Servings: 12

Ingredients:

Crabmeat, chopped – 1 pound

Chopped white onion – 2 tablespoons

Minced garlic – 1 tablespoon

Lemon juice – 2 tablespoons

Cream cheese, cubed – 16 ounces

Avocado mayonnaise – 1/3 cup

Grape juice – 2 tablespoons

Directions:

Place all the ingredients for the dip in a medium bowl and stir until combined.

Divide dip evenly between small bowls and serve as a party dip.

Nutrition:

Calories: 100, Fat: 4, Fiber: 1, Carbs: 4, Protein: 4

Creamy Cheddar and Bacon Spread with Almonds

Preparation Time: 10 minutes

Cooking Time: 10 minutes

Servings: 12

Ingredients:

Bacon, cooked and chopped – 12 ounces

Chopped sweet red pepper – 2 tablespoons

Medium white onion, peeled and chopped – 1

Salt – ¾ teaspoon

Ground black pepper – ½ teaspoon

Almonds, chopped – ½ cup

Cheddar cheese, grated – 1 pound

Avocado mayonnaise – 2 cups

Directions:

Place all the Ingredients for the dip in a medium bowl and stir until combined.

Divide dip evenly between small bowls and serve as a party dip.

Nutrition:

Calories: 184, Fat: 12, Fiber: 1, Carbs: 4,

Protein: 5

Green Tabasco Devilled Eggs

Preparation Time: 20 minutes

Cooking Time: 10 minutes

Servings: 6

Ingredients:

6 Eggs

1/3 cup Mayonnaise

1 ½ tbsp Green Tabasco

Salt and Pepper, to taste

Directions:

Place the eggs in a saucepan over medium heat and pour boiling water over, enough to cover them.

Cook for 6-8 minutes.

Place in an ice bath to cool.

When safe to handle, peel the eggs and slice them in half.

Scoop out the yolks and place them in a bowl.

Add the remaining ingredients.

Whisk to combine.

Fill the egg holes with the mixture.

Serve and enjoy!

Nutrition:

Calories 175

Total Fats 17g

Net Carbs: 5g

Protein 6g

Fiber: 1g

Herbed Cheese Balls

Preparation Time: 30 MIN

Cooking Time: 10 minutes

Servings: 20

Ingredients:

1/3 cup grated Parmesan Cheese

3 tbsp Heavy Cream

4 tbsp Butter, melted

¼ tsp Pepper

2 Eggs

1 cup Almond Flour

¼ cup Basil Leaves

¼ cup Parsley Leaves

2 tbsp chopped Cilantro Leaves

1/3 cup crumbled Feta Cheese

Directions:

Place the ingredients in your food processor.

Pulse until the mixture becomes smooth.

Transfer to a bowl and freeze for 20 minutes or so to set.

Shale the mixture into 20 balls.

Meanwhile, preheat the oven to 350 degrees F.

Arrange the cheese balls on a lined baking sheet.

Place in the oven and bake for 10 minutes.

Serve and enjoy!

Nutrition:

Calories 60 Total Fats 5g

Net Carbs: 8g Protein 2g

Fiber: 1g

Cheesy Salami Snack

Preparation Time: 30 MIN

Cooking Time: 10 minutes

Servings: 6

Ingredients: ¼ cup chopped Parsley

4 ounces Cream Cheese - 7 ounces dried Salami

Directions:

Preheat the oven to 325 degrees F. Slice the salami thinly (I got 30 slices).

Arrange the salami on a lined sheet and bake for 15 minutes. Arrange on a serving platter and top each salami slice with a bit of cream cheese. Serve and enjoy!

Nutrition:

Calories 139 Total Fats 15g

Net Carbs: 1g Protein 9g Fiber: 0g

Pesto & Olive Fat Bombs

Preparation Time: 25 MIN

Cooking Time: 10 minutes

Servings: 8

Ingredients: 2 tbsp Pesto Sauce

1 cup Cream Cheese - 10 Olives, sliced

½ cup grated Parmesan Cheese

Directions:

Place all of the ingredients in a bowl. Stir well to combine. Place in the freezer and freeze for 15-20 minutes to set. Shape into 8 balls. Serve and enjoy!

Nutrition:

Calories 123 Total Fats 13g Net Carbs: 3g

Protein 4g Fiber: 3g

Cheesy Broccoli Nuggets

Preparation Time: 25 MIN

Cooking Time: 10 minutes

Servings: 4

Ingredients:

1 cup shredded Cheese

¼ cup Almond Flour

2 cups Broccoli Florets, steamed in the microwave for 5 minutes

2 Egg Whites

Salt and Pepper, to taste

Directions:

Preheat the oven to 350 degrees F.

Place the broccoli florets in a bowl and mash them with a potato masher.

Add the remaining **Ingredients:** and mix well with your hands until combined.

Line a baking sheet with parchment paper.

Drop 20 scoops of the mixture onto the sheet.

Place in the oven and bake for 20 minutes or until golden.

Serve and enjoy!

Nutrition:

Calories 145

Total Fats 9g

Net Carbs: 4g

Protein 10g

Fiber: 1g

Salmon Fat Bombs

Preparation Time: 90 MIN

Cooking Time: 50 minutes

Servings: 6

Ingredients:

½ cup Cream Cheese

1 ½ tbsp chopped Dill

1 ¾ ounce Smoked Salmon, sliced

1 tbsp Lemon Juice

1/3 cup butter

¼ tsp Red Pepper Flakes

¼ tsp Garlic Powder

Pinch of Salt

¼ tsp Pepper

Directions:

Place the butter, salmon, lemon juice, and cream cheese in your food processor.

Add the seasonings.

Pulse until smooth.

Drop spoonfuls of the mixture onto a lined dish.

Sprinkle with the dill.

Place in the fridge for about 80 minutes.

Serve and enjoy!

Nutrition:

Calories 145

Total Fats 16g

Net Carbs: 7g

Protein 3g

Fiber: 1g

Guacamole Bacon Bombs

Preparation Time: 30 MIN

Cooking Time: 10 minutes

Servings: 6

Ingredients:

1 tsp minced Garlic

¼ cup Butter

½ Avocado, flesh scooped out

1 tbsp Lime Juice

1 tbsp chopped Cilantro

4 Bacon Slices, cooked and crumbled

3 tbsp diced Shallots

Salt and Pepper, to taste

1 tbsp minced Jalapeno

Directions:

Place all of the ingredients, except the bacon, in your food processor.

Pulse until smooth. Alternatively, you can do this by whisking in a bowl. Just keep in mind that this way, you will have chunks of garlic and jalapenos.

Transfer to a bowl and place in the freezer.

Freeze for 20 minutes, or until set.

Shape into 6 balls.

Coat them with bacon pieces.

Serve and enjoy!

Nutrition:

Calories 155

Total Fats 15g

Net Carbs: 4g

Protein 4g

Fiber: 3g

Fluffy Bites

Preparation Time: 20 minutes

Cooking Time: 60 minutes

Servings: 12

Ingredients:

2 Teaspoons Cinnamon

2/3 Cup Sour Cream

2 Cups Heavy Cream

1 Teaspoon Scraped Vanilla Bean

¼ Teaspoon Cardamom

4 Egg Yolks

Stevia to Taste

Directions:

Start by whisking your egg yolks until creamy and smooth.

Get out a double boiler, and add your eggs with the rest of your ingredients. Mix well.

Remove from heat, allowing it to cool until it reaches room temperature.

Refrigerate for an hour before whisking well.

Pour into molds, and freeze for at least an hour before serving.

Nutrition:

Calories: 363

Protein: 2

Fat: 40

Carbohydrates: 1

Coconut Fudge

Preparation Time: 20 minutes

Cooking Time: 60 minutes

Servings: 12

Ingredients:

2 Cups Coconut Oil

½ Cup Dark Cocoa Powder

½ Cup Coconut Cream

¼ Cup Almonds, Chopped

¼ Cup Coconut, Shredded

1 Teaspoon Almond Extract

Pinch of Salt

Stevia to Taste

Directions:

Pour your coconut oil and coconut cream in a bowl, whisking with an electric beater until smooth. Once the mixture becomes smooth and glossy, do not continue.

Begin to add in your cocoa powder while mixing slowly, making sure that there aren't any lumps.

Add in the rest of your ingredients, and mix well.

Line a bread pan with parchment paper, and freeze until it sets.

Slice into squares before serving.

Nutrition:

Calories: 172

Fat: 20

Carbohydrates: 3

Nutmeg Nougat

Preparation Time: 30 minutes

Cooking Time: 60 minutes

Servings: 12

Ingredients:

1 Cup Heavy Cream

1 Cup Cashew Butter

1 Cup Coconut, Shredded

½ Teaspoon Nutmeg

1 Teaspoon Vanilla Extract, Pure

Stevia to Taste

Directions:

Melt your cashew butter using a double boiler, and then stir in your vanilla extract, dairy cream, nutmeg and stevia. Make sure it's mixed well.

Remove from heat, allowing it to cool down before refrigerating it for a half-hour.

Shape into balls, and coat with shredded coconut. Chill for at least two hours before serving.

Nutrition:

Calories: 341 Fat: 34 Carbohydrates: 5

Sweet Almond Bites

Preparation Time: 30 minutes

Cooking Time: 90 minutes

Servings: 12

Ingredients:

18 Ounces Butter, Grass-Fed

2 Ounces Heavy Cream

½ Cup Stevia

2/3 Cup Cocoa Powder

1 Teaspoon Vanilla Extract, Pure

4 Tablespoons Almond Butter

Direction:

Use a double boiler to melt your butter before adding in all of your remaining ingredients.

Place the mixture into molds, freezing for two hours before serving.

Nutrition:

Calories: 350 Protein: 2 Fat: 38

Strawberry Cheesecake Minis

Preparation Time: 30 minutes

Cooking Time: 120 minutes

Servings: 12

Ingredients:

1 Cup Coconut Oil

1 Cup Coconut Butter

½ Cup Strawberries, Sliced

½ Teaspoon Lime Juice

2 Tablespoons Cream Cheese, Full Fat

Stevia to Taste

Directions:

Blend your strawberries.

Soften your cream cheese, and then add in your coconut butter.

Combine all **Ingredients:** together, and then pour your mixture into silicone molds.

Freeze for at least two hours before serving.

Nutrition:

Calories: 372 Protein: 1 Fat: 41

Carbohydrates: 2

Cocoa Brownies

Preparation Time: 10 minutes

Cooking Time: 30 minutes

Servings: 12

Ingredients:

1 Egg

2 Tablespoons Butter, Grass-Fed

2 Teaspoons Vanilla Extract, Pure

¼ Teaspoon Baking Powder

¼ Cup Cocoa Powder

1/3 Cup Heavy Cream

¾ Cup Almond Butter

Pinch Sea Salt

Directions:

Break your egg into a bowl, whisking until smooth.

Add in all of your wet ingredients, mixing well.

Mix all dry Ingredients into a bowl.

Sift your dry Ingredients into your wet ingredients, mixing to form a batter.

Get out a baking pan, greasing it before pouring in your mixture.

Heat your oven to 350 and bake for twenty-five minutes.

Allow it to cool before slicing and serve room temperature or warm.

Nutrition:

Calories: 184

Protein: 1

Fat: 20

Carbohydrates: 1

Chocolate Orange Bites

Preparation Time: 20 minutes

Cooking Time: 120 minutes

Servings: 6

Ingredients:

10 Ounces Coconut Oil

4 Tablespoons Cocoa Powder

¼ Teaspoon Blood Orange Extract

Stevia to Taste

Directions:

Melt half of your coconut oil using a double boiler, and then add in your stevia and orange extract.

Get out candy molds, pouring the mixture into it. Fill each mold halfway, and then place in the fridge until they set.

Melt the other half of your coconut oil, stirring in your cocoa powder and stevia, making sure that the mixture is smooth with no lumps.

Pour into your molds, filling them up all the way, and then allow it to set in the fridge before serving.

Nutrition:

Calories: *188*

Protein: *1*

Fat: 21

Carbohydrates: 5

Caramel Cones

Preparation Time: 25 minutes

Cooking Time: 120 minutes

Servings: 6

Ingredients:

2 Tablespoons Heavy Whipping Cream

2 Tablespoons Sour Cream

1 Tablespoon Caramel Sugar

1 Teaspoon Sea Salt, Fine

1/3 Cup Butter, Grass Fed

1/3 Cup Coconut Oil

Stevia to Taste

Directions:

Soften your coconut oil and butter, mixing.

Mix all ingredients to form a batter, and then place them in molds.

Top with a little salt, and keep refrigerated until serving.

Nutrition:

Calories: *100*

Fat: 12 Grams

Carbohydrates: 1

CHAPTER 24:

Poultry and eggs Recipes

Egg Butter

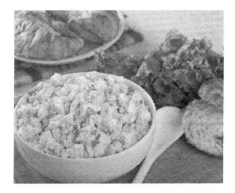

Preparation Time: 5 minutes;

Cooking Time: 0 minutes;

Servings: 2

Ingredients:

2 large eggs, hard-boiled

3-ounce unsalted butter ½ tsp dried oregano

½ tsp dried basil 2 leaves of iceberg lettuce

Seasoning:

½ tsp of sea salt

¼ tsp ground black pepper

Directions:

Peel the eggs, then chop them finely and place in a medium bowl. Add remaining **Ingredients:** and stir well. Serve egg butter wrapped in a lettuce leaf.

Nutrition:

159 Calories; Fats; 3 g Protein; 0.2 g

Net Carb; 0 g

Omelet

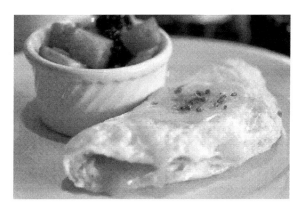

Preparation Time: 5 minutes

Cooking Time: 10 minutes;

Servings: 2

Ingredients:

2 eggs

2 tbsp shredded parmesan cheese, divided

1 tbsp unsalted butter

2 slices of turkey bacon, diced

Seasoning:

¼ tsp salt

1/8 tsp ground black pepper

Directions:

Crack eggs in a bowl, add salt and black pepper, whisk well until fluffy and then whisk in 1 tbsp cheese until combined.

Take a medium skillet pan, add bacon slices on it, cook for 3 minutes until sauté, then pour in the egg mixture and cook for 4 minutes or until the omelet is almost firm.

Lower heat to medium-low level, sprinkle remaining cheese on top of the omelet, then fold the omelet and cook for 1 minute.

Slide the omelet to a plate, cut it in half, and serve immediately.

Nutrition:

114.5 Calories; 9.3 g Fats; 4 g Protein;

1 g Net Carb; 0.2 g Fiber;

Classic Deviled Eggs

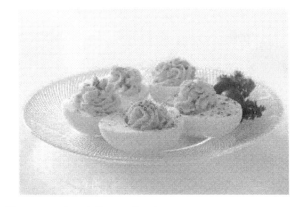

Preparation Time: 5 minutes

Cooking Time: 0 minutes;

Servings: 2

Ingredients:

2 eggs, boiled

1 1/3 tbsp mayonnaise

1/3 tsp mustard paste

¼ tsp apple cider vinegar

1/8 tsp paprika

Seasoning:

1/8 tsp salt

1/8 tsp ground black pepper

Directions:

Peel the boiled eggs, then slice in half lengthwise and transfer egg yolks to a medium bowl by using a spoon. Mash the egg yolk, add remaining ingredients except for paprika and stir until well combined. Pipe the egg yolk mixture into egg whites, then sprinkle with paprika and serve.

Nutrition: 145 Calories; 0.1 g Fiber;

12.8 g Fats; 6.9 g Protein; 0.7 g Net Carb;

Green Buttered Eggs

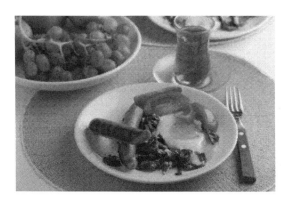

Preparation Time: 5 minutes

Cooking Time: 5 minutes;

Servings: 2

Ingredients:

¼ cup cilantro leaves, chopped

1/2 tsp minced garlic - ¼ cup parsley, chopped

1 tsp thyme leaves - 2 eggs

Seasoning: - ¼ tsp salt - ¼ tsp cayenne pepper

1 tbsp butter, unsalted - 1/2 tbsp avocado oil

Directions:

Take a medium skillet pan, place it over low heat, add oil and butter, and when the butter melts, add garlic and cook for 1 minute until fragrant. Add thyme, cook for 30 seconds until it begins to brown, then add cilantro and parsley, switch heat to medium level and then cook for 2 minutes until crisp. Cracks eggs on top of herbs, cover with a lid, then switch heat to the low level and cook for 2 to 3 minutes until yolks are set and cooked to the desired level. Serve.

Nutrition:

165 Calories; 14.4 g Fats; 7.3 g Protein;

0.9 g Net Carb; 0.4 g Fiber;

Egg Salad

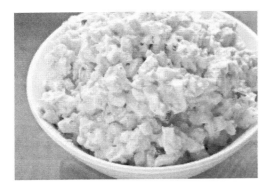

Preparation Time: 5 minutes

Cooking Time: 0 minutes

Servings: 2

Ingredients: Seasoning:

2 tbsp mayonnaise - 1 tsp lemon juice

2 large eggs, hard-boiled

2 slices of bacon, cooked, crumbled

1/8 tsp cracked black pepper - ¼ tsp salt

Directions:

Peel the eggs, then dice them and place them in a bowl. Add remaining ingredients except for bacon and stir until well mixed. Top with bacon and serve.

Nutrition:

240.3 Calories; 10g Fats; 10.8 g Protein;

0 g Net Carb; 0 g Fiber;

Pesto Scramble

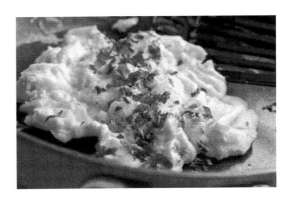

Preparation Time: 5 minutes

Cooking Time: 5 minutes

Servings: 2

Ingredients:

2 eggs

2 tbsp grated cheddar cheese

1 tbsp unsalted butter - 1 tbsp basil pesto

Seasoning:

1/8 tsp salt

1/8 tsp ground black pepper

Directions:

Crack eggs in a bowl, add cheese, black pepper, salt, and pesto and whisk until combined.

Take a skillet pan, place it over medium heat, add butter and when it melts, pour in the egg mixture, and cook for 3 to 5 minutes until eggs have scrambled to the desired level. Serve.

Nutrition:

159.5 Calories; 14.5 g Fats;

7 g Protein; 0.4 g Net Carb; 0.1 g Fiber;

Fried Eggs

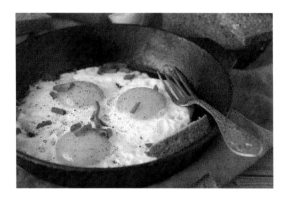

Preparation Time: 5 minutes

Cooking Time: 8 minutes

Servings: 2

Ingredients:

2 eggs

2 tbsp unsalted butter

Seasoning:

¼ tsp salt

1/8 tsp ground black pepper

Directions:

Take a skillet pan, place it over medium heat, add butter and when it has melted, crack eggs in the pan.

Cook eggs for 3 to 5 minutes until fried to the desired level, then transfer the eggs to serving plates and sprinkle with salt and black pepper.

Serve.

Nutrition:

179 Calories; 16.5 g Fats;

7.6 g Protein; 0 g Net Carb; 0 g Fiber;

Chicken and Bacon Pancake

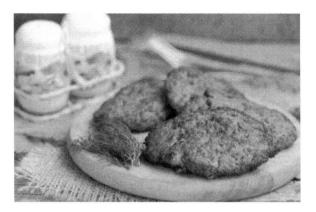

Preparation Time: 5 minutes

Cooking Time: 8 minutes

Servings: 2

Ingredients:

1 chicken thigh, debone

2 slices of bacon

1 egg

2 tbsp coconut oil

Seasoning:

¼ tsp salt

1/8 tsp ground black pepper

Directions:

Cut chicken into bite-size pieces, place them in a food processor, add bacon, egg, salt, and black pepper and process until well combined.

Take a frying pan, place it over medium heat, add 1 tbsp oil and when hot, scoop chicken mixture in the pan, shape each scoop into a round pancake and cook for 4 minutes per side until brown and cooked. When done, transfer pancakes into a plate, drizzle with remaining oil and serve.

Nutrition:

222 Calories; 17 g Fats; 16.5 g Protein;

0 g Net Carb;0 g Fiber;

Egg and Cheese Breakfast

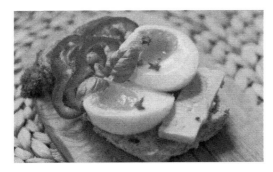

Preparation Time: 20 minutes

Cooking Time: 5 minutes

Servings: 2

Ingredients:

2 large eggs

2 blocks of cheddar cheese, each about 1-ounce

Directions:

Take a medium saucepan, half full with water, add eggs in it, then place the pan over medium heat and bring to boil, covering with the lid.

When water starts boiling, remove the pan from heat and let it rest until eggs have cooked to the desired level, 4 minutes for the runny center, 6 minutes for the semi-soft center, 10 minutes for medium, and 16 minutes for hard-boiled.

Then drain the eggs, rinse it under cold water until cooled, and then peel them.

Serve eggs with cheese.

Nutrition:

271 Calories; 21.5 g Fats; 17.6 g Protein;

1.1 g Net Carb; 0 g Fiber;

Eggs in Clouds

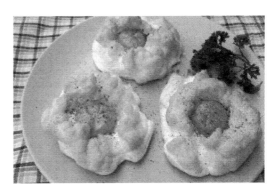

Preparation Time: 5 minutes

Cooking Time: 5 minutes

Servings: 2

Ingredients:

2 eggs

2 tbsp chopped bacon, cooked

Seasoning:

¼ tsp salt

1/8 tsp ground black pepper

Directions:

Turn on the oven, then set it to 350 degrees F and let it preheat.

Separate egg whites and yolks between two bowls, and then beat the egg whites until stiff peaks form.

Add bacon, fold until mixed, scoop the mixture into two mounds onto a baking sheet lined with parchment paper.

Make a small well in the middle of each mound by using a small bowl, bake for 3 minutes, then add an egg yolk into each well and continue baking for 2 minutes. Season eggs with salt and black pepper and then serve.

Nutrition:

101 Calories; 7.1 g Fats; 8.6 g Protein;

0.8 g Net Carb; 0 g Fiber;

Buttery Scrambled Eggs

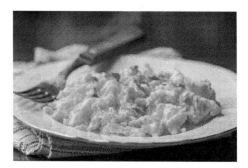

Preparation Time: 5 minutes

Cooking Time: 6 minutes

Servings: 2

Ingredients:

3 eggs

¼ tsp salt

1/8 tsp ground black pepper

2 tbsp chopped unsalted butter, cold

1 tbsp unsalted butter, softened

Directions:

Take a bowl, cracked eggs in it, whisk until well combined and then stir in chopped cold butter until mixed.

Take a skillet pan, place it over medium-low heat, add butter and when it melts, pour in the egg mixture and cook for 1 minute, don't stir.

Then stir the omelet and cook for 1 to 2 minutes until thoroughly cooked and scramble to the desired level.

Season scramble eggs with salt and black pepper and then serve.

Nutrition:

81.5 Calories;

3.75 g Fats; 3.75 g Protein;

0.25 g Net Carb; 0 g Fiber;

Cream Cheese Pancakes

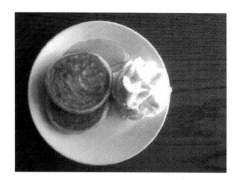

Preparation Time: 5 minutes

Cooking Time: 5 minutes

Servings: 2

Ingredients:

2 oz cream cheese

2 eggs

½ tsp cinnamon

1 tsp unsalted butter

Directions:

Place cream cheese in a blender, add eggs and cinnamon, pulse for 1 minute or until smooth, and then let the batter rest for 5 minutes.

Take a skillet pan, place it over medium heat, add butter and when it melts, drop one-fourth of the batter into the pan, spread evenly, and cook the pancakes for 2 minutes per side until done.

Transfer pancakes to a plate and serve.

Nutrition:

97.8 Calories;

8.4 g Fats;

4.4 g Protein;

1 g Net Carb;

0.2 g Fiber;

Sheet Pan Eggs with Bell Pepper and Chives

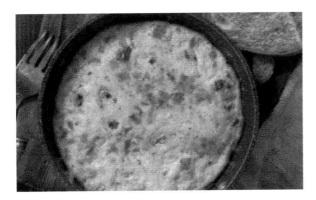

Preparation Time: 5 minutes

Cooking Time: 8 minutes

Servings: 2

Ingredients:

½ of medium red bell pepper, chopped

2 tbsp chopped chives

2 eggs

Seasoning:

¼ tsp salt

1/8 tsp ground black pepper

Directions:

Turn on the oven, then set it to 350 degrees F and let it preheat.

Meanwhile, crack eggs in a bowl, add remaining ingredients and whisk until combined.

Take a small heatproof dish, pour in egg mixture, and bake for 5 to 8 minutes until set.

When done, cut it into two squares and then serve.

Nutrition:

87 Calories; 5.4 g Fats;

7.2 g Protein; 1.7 g Net Carb;

0.7 g Fiber;

Crepe

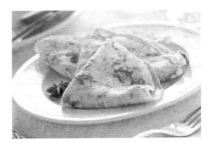

Preparation Time: 5 minutes

Cooking Time: 9 minutes

Servings: 2

Ingredients:

2/3 tbsp psyllium husk

1 1/3 tbsp cream cheese

2 eggs

1 egg white

1 tbsp unsalted butter

Directions:

Prepare the batter and for this, place all the ingredients in a bowl, except for butter, and then whisk by using a stick blender until smooth and very liquid.

Take a skillet pan, place it over medium heat, add ½ tbsp butter and when it melts, pour in half of the batter, spread evenly, and cook until the top has firmed.

Carefully flip the crepe, then continue cooking for 2 minutes until cooked and then transfer it to a plate.

Add remaining butter and when it melts, cook another crepe in the same manner and then serve.

Nutrition:

118 Calories; 9.4 g Fats;

6.5 g Protein; 1 g Net Carb;

0.9 g Fiber;

Omelet with Meat

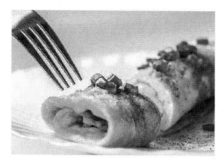

Preparation Time: 5 minutes

Cooking Time: 12 minutes

Servings: 2

 Ingredients:

2 oz ground turkey

1 tbsp chopped spinach

1 tbsp whipped topping

2 eggs

2 tbsp grated mozzarella cheese

Seasoning:

¼ tsp salt

1/8 tsp ground black pepper

Directions:

Take a skillet pan, place it over medium heat, add ground turkey and cook for 5 minutes until cooked through.

Meanwhile, crack eggs in a bowl, add whipped topping and spinach and whisk until combined.

When the meat is cooked, transfer it to a plate, then switch heat to the low level and pour in the egg mixture.

Cook the eggs for 3 minutes until the bottom is firm, then flip it and cook for 3 minutes until the omelet is firmed, covering the pan.

Sprinkle cheese on the omelet, cook for 1 minute until cheese has melted, and then slide omelet to a plate.

Spread ground meat on the omelet, roll it, then cut it in half and serve.

Nutrition:

126.3 Calories;

8.6 g Fats;

10.7 g Protein;

1.5 g Net Carb;

0 g Fiber;

CHAPTER 25:

Meat Recipes

Beef with Cabbage Noodles

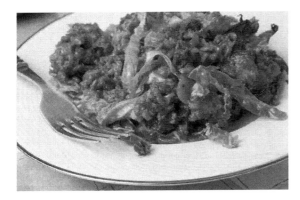

Preparation Time: 5 minutes

Cooking Time: 18 minutes

Servings: 2

Ingredients:

4 oz ground beef

1 cup chopped cabbage

4 oz tomato sauce

½ tsp minced garlic

½ cup of water

Seasoning:

½ tbsp coconut oil

½ tsp salt

¼ tsp Italian seasoning

1/8 tsp dried basil

Directions:

Take a skillet pan, place it over medium heat, add oil and when hot, add beef and cook for 5 minutes until nicely browned.

Meanwhile, prepare the cabbage and for it slice the cabbage into thin shred.

When the beef has cooked, add garlic, season with salt, basil, and Italian seasoning, stir well and continue cooking for 3 minutes until meat has thoroughly cooked.

Pour in tomato sauce and water, stir well and bring the mixture to boil.

Then reduce heat to medium-low level, add cabbage, stir well until well mixed and simmer for 3 to 5 minutes until cabbage is softened, covering the pan.

Uncover the pan and continue simmering the beef until most of the cooking liquid has evaporated.

Serve.

Nutrition:

188.5 Calories;

12.5 g Fats;

15.5 g Protein;

2.5 g Net Carb;

1 g Fiber;

Roast Beef and Mozzarella Plate

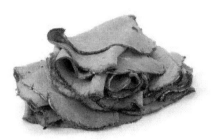

Preparation Time: 5 minutes

Cooking Time: 0 minutes;

Servings: 2

Ingredients:

4 slices of roast beef

½ ounce chopped lettuce

1 avocado, pitted

2 oz mozzarella cheese, cubed

½ cup mayonnaise

Seasoning:

¼ tsp salt

1/8 tsp ground black pepper

2 tbsp avocado oil

Directions:

Scoop out flesh from the avocado and divide it evenly between two plates.

Add slices of roast beef, lettuce, and cheese and then sprinkle with salt and black pepper.

Serve with avocado oil and mayonnaise.

Nutrition:

267.7 Calories; 24.5 g Fats;

9.5 g Protein; 1.5 g Net Carb;

2 g Fiber;

Beef and Broccoli

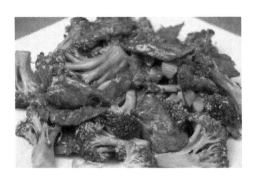

Preparation Time: 5 minutes

Cooking Time: 10 minutes;

Servings: 2

Ingredients:

6 slices of beef roast, cut into strips

1 scallion, chopped

3 oz broccoli florets, chopped

1 tbsp avocado oil - 1 tbsp butter, unsalted

Seasoning: - ¼ tsp salt

1/8 tsp ground black pepper

1 ½ tbsp soy sauce - 3 tbsp chicken broth

Directions:

Take a medium skillet pan, place it over medium heat, add oil and when hot, add beef strips and cook for 2 minutes until hot. Transfer beef to a plate, add scallion to the pan, then add butter and cook for 3 minutes until tender.

Add remaining ingredients, stir until mixed, switch heat to the low level and simmer for 3 to 4 minutes until broccoli is tender.

Return beef to the pan, stir until well combined and cook for 1 minute.

Serve.

Nutrition:

245 Calories; 15.7 g Fats; 21.6 g Protein;

1.7 g Net Carb; 1.3 g Fiber;

Garlic Herb Beef Roast

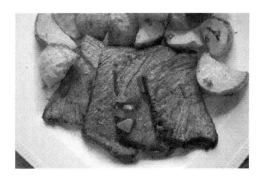

Preparation Time: 5 minutes

Cooking Time: 10 minutes;

Servings: 2

Ingredients:

6 slices of beef roast

½ tsp garlic powder

1/3 tsp dried thyme

¼ tsp dried rosemary

2 tbsp butter, unsalted

Seasoning:

1/3 tsp salt

1/4 tsp ground black pepper

Directions:

Prepare the spice mix and for this, take a small bowl, place garlic powder, thyme, rosemary, salt, and black pepper and then stir until mixed.

Sprinkle spice mix on the beef roast.

Take a medium skillet pan, place it over medium heat, add butter and when it melts, add beef roast and then cook for 5 to 8 minutes until golden brown and cooked.

Serve.

Nutrition:

140 Calories; 12.7 g Fats; 5.5 g Protein;

0.1 g Net Carb; 0.2 g Fiber;

Sprouts Stir-fry with Kale, Broccoli, and Beef

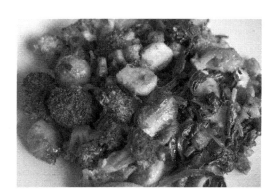

Preparation Time: 5 minutes

Cooking Time: 8 minutes;

Servings: 2

Ingredients:

3 slices of beef roast, chopped

2 oz Brussels sprouts, halved

4 oz broccoli florets - 3 oz kale

1 ½ tbsp butter, unsalted

1/8 tsp red pepper flakes

Seasoning:

¼ tsp garlic powder - ¼ tsp salt

1/8 tsp ground black pepper

Directions:

Take a medium skillet pan, place it over medium heat, add ¾ tbsp butter and when it melts, add broccoli florets and sprouts, sprinkle with garlic powder, and cook for 2 minutes. Season vegetables with salt and red pepper flakes, add chopped beef, stir until mixed and continue cooking for 3 minutes until browned on one side.

Then add kale along with remaining butter, flip the vegetables and cook for 2 minutes until kale leaves wilts. Serve.

Nutrition: 125 Calories; 9.4 g Fats;

4.8 g Protein; 1.7 g Net Carb; 2.6 g Fiber;

Beef and Vegetable Skillet

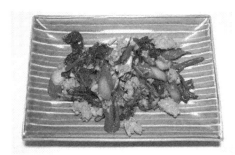

Preparation Time: 5 minutes

Cooking Time: 15 minutes

Servings: 2

Ingredients:

3 oz spinach, chopped

½ pound ground beef

2 slices of bacon, diced

2 oz chopped asparagus

Seasoning:

3 tbsp coconut oil

2 tsp dried thyme

2/3 tsp salt

½ tsp ground black pepper

Directions:

Take a skillet pan, place it over medium heat, add oil and when hot, add beef and bacon and cook for 5 to 7 minutes until slightly browned.

Then add asparagus and spinach, sprinkle with thyme, stir well and cook for 7 to 10 minutes until thoroughly cooked.

Season skillet with salt and black pepper and serve.

Nutrition:

332.5 Calories; 26 g Fats; 23.5 g Protein;

1.5 g Net Carb; 1 g Fiber;

Beef, Pepper and Green Beans Stir-fry

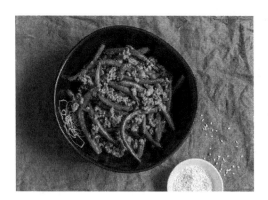

Preparation Time: 5 minutes;

Cooking Time: 18 minutes

Servings: 2

Ingredients:

6 oz ground beef

2 oz chopped green bell pepper

4 oz green beans

3 tbsp grated cheddar cheese

Seasoning:

½ tsp salt - ¼ tsp ground black pepper

¼ tsp paprika

Directions:

Take a skillet pan, place it over medium heat, add ground beef and cook for 4 minutes until slightly browned. Then add bell pepper and green beans, season with salt, paprika, and black pepper, stir well and continue cooking for 7 to 10 minutes until beef and vegetables have cooked through. Sprinkle cheddar cheese on top, then transfer pan under the broiler and cook for 2 minutes until cheese has melted and the top is golden brown. Serve.

Nutrition:

282.5 Calories; 17.6 g Fats; 26.1 g Protein;

2.9 g Net Carb; 2.1 g Fiber;

Cheesy Meatloaf

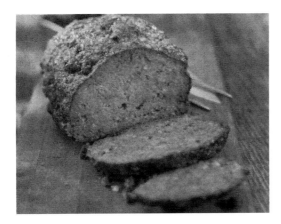

Preparation Time: 5 minutes

Cooking Time: 4 minutes

Servings: 2

Ingredients:

4 oz ground turkey

1 egg

1 tbsp grated mozzarella cheese

¼ tsp Italian seasoning

½ tbsp soy sauce

Seasoning:

¼ tsp salt

1/8 tsp ground black pepper

Directions:

Take a bowl, place all the Ingredients in it, and stir until mixed. Take a heatproof mug, spoon in prepared mixture and microwave for 3 minutes at high heat setting until cooked. When done, let meatloaf rest in the mug for 1 minute, then take it out, cut it into two slices and serve.

Nutrition:

196.5 Calories; 13.5 g Fats; 18.7 g Protein;

18.7 g Net Carb; 0 g Fiber;

Roast Beef and Vegetable Plate

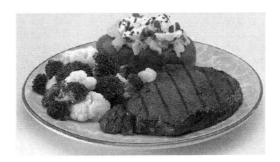

Preparation Time: 10 minutes

Cooking Time: 10 minutes;

Servings: 2

Ingredients:

2 scallions, chopped in large pieces

1 ½ tbsp coconut oil

4 thin slices of roast beef

4 oz cauliflower and broccoli mix

1 tbsp butter, unsalted

Seasoning:

1/2 tsp salt - 1/3 tsp ground black pepper

1 tsp dried parsley

Directions:

Turn on the oven, then set it to 400 degrees F, and let it preheat. Take a baking sheet, grease it with oil, place slices of roast beef on one side, and top with butter. Take a separate bowl, add cauliflower and broccoli mix, add scallions, drizzle with oil, season with remaining salt and black pepper, toss until coated and then spread vegetables on the empty side of the baking sheet.

Bake for 5 to 7 minutes until beef is nicely browned and vegetables are tender-crisp, tossing halfway. Distribute beef and vegetables between two plates and then serve.

Nutrition: 313 Calories; 26 g Fats;

15.6 g Protein; 2.8 g Net Carb; 1.9 g Fiber;

Steak and Cheese Plate

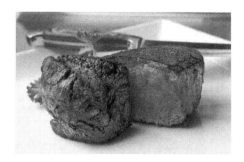

Preparation Time: 5 minutes;

Cooking Time: 10 minutes;

Servings: 2

Ingredients:

1 green onion, chopped

2 oz chopped lettuce

2 beef steaks

2 oz of cheddar cheese, sliced

½ cup mayonnaise

Seasoning:

¼ tsp salt

1/8 tsp ground black pepper

3 tbsp avocado oil

Directions:

Prepare the steak, and for this, season it with salt and black pepper.

Take a medium skillet pan, place it over medium heat, add oil and when hot, add seasoned steaks and cook for 7 to 10 minutes until cooked to the desired level. When done, distribute steaks between two plates, add scallion, lettuce, and cheese slices. Drizzle with remaining oil and then serve with mayonnaise.

Nutrition:

714 Calories; 65.3 g Fats; 25.3 g Protein;

4 g Net Carb; 5.3 g Fiber;

Garlicky Steaks with Rosemary

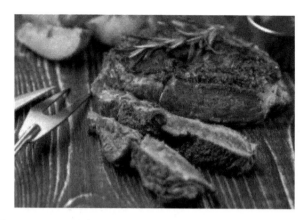

Preparation Time: 25 minutes

Cooking Time: 12 minutes;

Servings: 2

Ingredients:

2 beef steaks - 1/4 of a lime, juiced

1 ½ tsp garlic powder - ¾ tsp dried rosemary

2 ½ tbsp avocado oil

Seasoning:

½ tsp salt - ¼ tsp ground black pepper

Directions:

Prepare steaks, and for this, sprinkle garlic powder on all sides of steak. Take a shallow dish, place 1 ½ tbsp oil and lime juice in it, whisk until combined, add steaks, turn to coat and let it marinate for 20 minutes at room temperature. Then take a griddle pan, place it over medium-high heat and grease it with remaining oil. Season marinated steaks with salt and black pepper, add to the griddle pan and cook for 7 to 12 minutes until cooked to the desired level.

When done, wrap steaks in foil for 5 minutes, then cut into slices across the grain.

Sprinkle rosemary over steaks slices and then serve.

Nutrition: 213 Calories; 13 g Fats;

22 g Protein; 1 g Net Carb; 0 g Fiber;

CHAPTER 26:

Seafood and Fish Recipes

Herb Baked Salmon Fillets

Preparation Time: 35 MIN

Cooking Time: 18 minutes

Servings: 6

Ingredients:

2 lbs. salmon fillets

1/2 cup chopped fresh mushrooms

1/2 cup chopped green onions

4 oz. butter

4 Tbsp coconut oil

1/2 cup tamari soy sauce

1 tsp minced garlic

1/4 tsp thyme

1/2 tsp rosemary

1/4 tsp tarragon

1/2 tsp ground ginger

1/2 tsp basil

1 tsp oregano leaves

Directions:

Preheat oven to 350 degrees F. Line a large baking pan with foil.

Cut salmon filet into pieces. Put the salmon into the Ziploc bag with the tamari sauce, sesame oil, and spices sauce mixture. Refrigerate the salmon and marinate it for 4 hours.

Put the salmon in a baking pan and bake fillets for 10-15 minutes.

Melt the butter. Add the chopped fresh mushrooms and green onion to it, and mix. Remove the salmon from the oven, and pour the butter mixture over the salmon fillets, making sure each fillet gets covered.

Bake for about 10 minutes more. Serve immediately.

Nutrition:

Calories 449 Total Fats 34g

Net Carbs: 7g Protein 33g

Fiber 7g

Salmon with a Walnut Crust

Preparation Time: 20 MIN

Cooking Time: 18 minutes

Servings: 2

Ingredients:

½ cup Walnuts

½ tbsp Dijon mustard

6 oz Salmon filets

Salt

2 tbsp Maple syrup, sugar-free

¼ tsp Dill

1 tbsp Olive oil

Directions:

Set oven to 350 F.

Put mustard, syrup, and walnuts into a processor and pulse until the mixture is pasty.

Heat oil in a pot and place the skin side down in the pan and sear for 3 minutes.

Top it with walnut blend and place into a lined baking dish.

Bake for 8 minutes.

Serve.

Nutrition:

Calories 373 Total Fats 43g

Net Carbs: 3g Protein 20g Fiber 1g

Baked Glazed Salmon

Preparation Time: 30 MIN

Cooking Time: 18 minutes

Servings: 2

Ingredients:

2 pcs salmon fillets

For the glaze:

1 tbsp sweet mustard

1 tbsp Dijon mustard - 1 tbsp lemon juice

½ tsp chili flakes

1 tsp sage

Salt to taste

1 tbsp olive oil

Directions:

Set the oven at 350 F.

In a bowl, whisk all the ingredients for the glaze.

Place the salmon fillets on a baking sheet lined with parchment paper and brush the salmon fillets with the glaze.

Place in the oven to bake for 20 minutes. Serve warm.

Nutrition:

Calories 379 Total Fats 29g Net Carbs: 3g

Protein 35g

Salmon Burgers

Preparation Time: 20 MIN

Cooking Time: 20 minutes

Servings: 4

Ingredients:

1 1oz can cook salmon flakes in water

2 organic eggs

1 cup gluten-free breadcrumbs

1 small onion, chopped

1 tbsp fresh parsley, chopped

3 tbsp mayonnaise - 2 tsp lemon juice

Salt to taste

1 tbsp olive oil

1 tbsp ghee

Directions:

Crack the eggs into a bowl and use a hand mixer to whisk them until fluffy.

Add the bread crumbs in the bowl with the egg and combine well.

Add the onions, parsley, and mayonnaise and mix again.

Add the salmon flakes, and drizzle the lemon juice and olive oil. Season with salt and stir again.

Divide the mixture into 4 parts and then create patties using your hands.

Heat the ghee in a cast-iron skillet over the medium-high fire and fry the patties until golden brown.

Serve with a salad on the side.

Nutrition:

Calories 281

Total Fats 22g

Net Carbs: 1g

Protein 2g

Fiber 8g

Keto Crab Sushi

Preparation Time: 20 MIN

Cooking Time: 20 minutes

Servings: 1

Ingredients:

1 ½ cup cauliflower florets, chopped

½ cup softened cream cheese

¾ cup crab meat, cooked

3 tbsp mayonnaise

1 tbsp Sriracha

1 pc Nori wrapper

Directions:

Pulse the cauliflower florets in a food processor and chop and until you achieve a rice-like texture.

Transfer the chopped cauliflower in a microwavable container and zap 5 minutes on high or until the vegetable is cooked.

Add the cream cheese with the hot cauliflower and stir. Place the mixture in the fridge and let it cool for an hour.

Place the nori wrapper on top of a sushi mat and spread the cauliflower mixture over it. Remember to leave a 1-inch border.

Meanwhile, combine all the remaining ingredients in a bowl and then scoop the crab mixture in the middle of the cauliflower rice.

Roll the sushi and cut into 6-8 pcs.

Nutrition:

Calories 446 Total Fats 35g

Net Carbs: 24g Protein 14g Fiber 8g

Coco Shrimps and Chili Dip

Preparation Time: 20 MIN

Cooking Time: 20 minutes

Servings: 2

Ingredients:

12 pcs large shrimps, peeled and deveined

1 ½ cup coconut shreds, unsweetened

¼ cup coconut flakes

6 tbsp mayonnaise

3 tbsp coconut milk

1 egg yolk

Olive oil for frying

For the dip

4 tbsp mayonnaise

2 tsp chili garlic sauce

1 tsp lime juice

Directions:

Pat the shrimp dry set aside.

Combine the coconut shreds, coconut flakes, mayo, coconut milk, and egg yolk. Stir well.

Place the shrimps with the coconut mixture. Make sure that the shrimps are well-coated with the variety.

Heat oil in the pan and fry the shrimps until golden brown.

Whisk all the ingredients of the dip in a small bowl. Serve alongside with the shrimps.

Nutrition:

Calories 670

Total Fats 60g

Net Carbs: 7g

Protein 11g

Fiber: 3g

Tuna/Smoked Salmon Salad

Preparation Time: 10 MIN

Cooking Time: 20 minutes

Servings: 2

Ingredients:

5 oz Smoked Salmon

1 Hard Boiled Egg

½ Avocados

1 cup green beans (Steamed)

5 cherry tomatoes

1 tbsp Red Onion

½ cup celery

Directions:

Place all ingredients into a bowl, mix and enjoy.

Nutrition:

Calories 270 Total Fats 19g Net Carbs: 26g

Protein 17g Fiber 4g

Salmon Salad in Avocado Cups

Preparation Time: 35 MIN

Cooking Time: 20 minutes

Servings: 2

Ingredients:

1 medium-sized salmon fillet

1 shallot, diced

¼ cup mayo - ½ juice of the lime

2 tsp fresh dill, chopped

1 tbsp ghee

1 large avocado, sliced in half and pitted

Salt and pepper to taste

Directions:

Preheat oven to 400 F.

Place the salmon fillet on a baking sheet and drizzle it with ghee and juice of a lime. Season with salt and pepper and place in the oven to cook for 20-25 minutes.

When done, allow the salmon to cook for a few minutes and shred using a fork.

Place the salmon in a bowl, add the diced shallot, and mix well.

Add the dill and mayo to the salmon mixture and combine well. Set aside.

Remove the insides of the avocado halves making sure that the skin is still intact to make cups.

Mash the avocado meat in a bowl and then add to the salmon mixture. Combine well.

Transfer the avocado and tuna salad back to the avocado cups and serve.

Nutrition:

Calories 463 Total Fats 35g Net Carbs: 4g

Protein 27g

Mackerel Salad

Preparation Time: 20 MIN

Cooking Time: 20 minutes

Servings: 2

Ingredients:

2 Eggs (organic) - 2 Cups Green beans

1 Tbsp Coconut oil - Black pepper

2 Mackerel filets (3 oz.) - 1 Avocado

4 Cups Mixed greens

¼ Tsp Salt

For dressing:

2 Tsp Lemon juice

1 Tsp Dijon mustard

2 Tbsp Olive oil (extra-virgin)

Directions:

Cook eggs until hard-boiled and then place them into a pan with cold water.

Fill a pot with water and add salt to taste. Cook beans for 5 minutes until crisp, drain and put aside until needed.

Use a knife to make diagonal slices along the skin of mackerel and use pepper and salt to season.

Heat coconut oil in a skillet and place mackerels with skin down into the pan. Cook for 5-7 minutes until the skin is crisp. Remove skillet from heat and put aside until needed.

Prepare the dressing by mixing all the ingredients. Slice eggs into quarters and rinse greens and drain.

Place greens into a bowl and top with mackerel and eggs; drizzle with dressing. Serve.

Nutrition:

Calories 609 Total Fats 49g Net Carbs: 11g

Protein 23g Fiber 5g

Crab Cakes

Preparation Time: 20 MIN

Cooking Time: 20 minutes

Servings: 6

Ingredients:

1 lb crabmeat

¼ cup parsley, chopped

1 tsp jalapeno pepper, seeds removed and chopped

1 tsp fresh lemon juice

½ tsp mustard powder

½ cup mayonnaise

2 tbsp olive oil

2 green onions, diced

¼ cup cilantro, diced

1 tsp Worcestershire sauce

1 tsp Old Bay seasoning

1 egg

Salt

Directions:

Sort crab and remove shell bits, transfer to a bowl and put aside.

Add parsley, jalapeno, lemon juice, mustard powder, green onion, cilantro, Worcestershire sauce and Old Bay seasoning. Gently fold mixture so that crab does not fall apart.

Add egg to a bowl and beat, then add mayo and combine. Add crab to the mayo mixture and place it in a strainer. Put a strainer in a bowl and wrap with plastic wrap; place in the refrigerator overnight.

Remove the strainer from the bowl and discard excess liquid. Shape crab cakes and cover in the refrigerator while the oven heats up.

Set oven to 200 F.

Heat 1 tbsp of oil in skillet and place 3 of crab cakes into the pan. Cook for 3 minutes until golden and firm, then flip and cook for 3 more minutes. Transfer to baking sheet and place in oven. Repeat with leftover crab cakes.

Serve.

Nutrition:

Calories 257

Total Fats 15g

Net Carbs: 6g

Protein 14g

Fiber: 3g

Shrimp & Avocado Salad

Preparation Time: 45 MIN

Cooking Time: 40 minutes

Servings: 2

Ingredients:

12 oz. shrimp, peel removed and deveined

One ripe avocado, peeled, cored, and cut into cubes

3 cups baby spinach

1 tomato, chopped

¼ cup green onions, chopped

¼ cup fresh cilantro, chopped

For the marinade:

4 tbsp olive oil

2 tbsp lime juice

Salt and pepper to taste

¼ tsp garlic powder

¼ tsp chili powder

Directions:

In a bowl, whisk all the ingredients for the marinade.

Add the shrimp into the bowl and toss. Allow marinating for 30 minutes in the fridge.

When the shrimps are ready, heat a non-stick pan over medium fire. Throw in the shrimp and cook for 2 minutes on each side.

Toss together the avocado cubes, baby spinach, chopped tomatoes, green onions, and cilantro in a bowl.

Top with the cooked shrimp and drizzle with an additional 1 tbsp of olive oil.

Nutrition:

Calories 428

Total Fats 28g

Net Carbs: 11g

Protein 45g

Fiber 5g

CHAPTER 27:

Smoothie Recipes

Matcha Green Juice

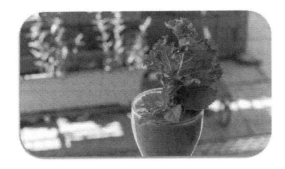

Preparation Time: 10 minutes

Cooking Time: 0 minutes

Servings: 2

Ingredients:

5 ounces fresh kale - 2 ounces fresh arugula

¼ cup fresh parsley

4 celery stalks

1 green apple, cored and chopped

1 (1-inch) piece fresh ginger, peeled

1 lemon, peeled

½ teaspoon matcha green tea

Directions

Add all ingredients into a juicer and extract the juice according to the manufacturer's method.

Pour into 2 glasses and serve immediately.

Nutrition: Calories: 113, Sodium: 22 mg,

Dietary Fibre: 1.2 g, Total Fat: 2.1 g,

Total Carbs: 12.3 g, Protein: 1.3 g.

Celery Juice

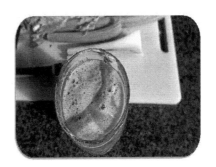

Preparation Time: 10 minutes

Cooking Time: 0 minutes

Servings: 2

Ingredients:

8 celery stalks with leaves

2 tablespoons fresh ginger, peeled

1 lemon, peeled

½ cup of filtered water

Pinch of salt

Instructions

Place all the ingredients in a blender and pulse until well combined.

Through a fine mesh strainer, strain the juice and transfer into 2 glasses.

Serve immediately.

Nutrition:

Calories: 32, Sodium: 21 mg, Dietary Fibre: 1.4 g,

Total Fat: 1.1 g, Total Carbs: 1.3 g, Protein: 1.2 g.

Kale & Orange Juice

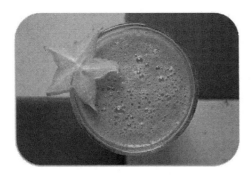

Preparation Time: 10 minutes

Cooking Time: 0 minutes

Servings: 2

Ingredients:

5 large oranges, peeled

2 bunches fresh kale

Directions

Add all ingredients into a juicer and extract the juice according to the manufacturer's method.

Pour into two glasses and serve immediately.

Nutrition:

Calories: 315,

Sodium: 34 mg,

Dietary Fibre: 1.3 g,

Total Fat: 4.1 g,

Total Carbs: 14.3 g,

Protein: 1.2 g.

Apple & Cucumber Juice

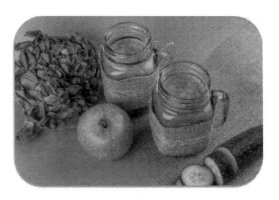

Preparation Time: 10 minutes

Cooking Time: 0 minutes

Servings: 2

Ingredients:

3 large apples, cored and sliced

2 large cucumbers, sliced

4 celery stalks

1 (1-inch) piece fresh ginger, peeled

1 lemon, peeled

Directions

Add all ingredients into a juicer and extract the juice according to the manufacturer's method.

Pour into 2 glasses and serve immediately.

Nutrition:

Calories: 230,

Sodium: 31 mg,

Dietary Fibre: 1.3 g,

Total Fat: 2.1 g,

Total Carbs: 1.3 g,

Protein: 1.2 g.

Lemony Green Juice

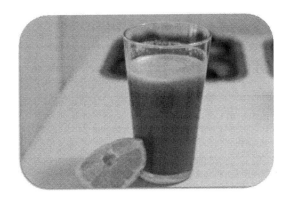

Preparation Time: 10 minutes

Cooking Time: 0 minutes

Servings: 2

Ingredients:

2 large green apples, cored and sliced

4 cups fresh kale leaves

4 tablespoons fresh parsley leaves

1 tablespoon fresh ginger, peeled

1 lemon, peeled

½ cup of filtered water

Pinch of salt

Directions

Place all the ingredients in a blender and pulse until well combined.

Through a fine mesh strainer, strain the juice and transfer into 2 glasses.

Serve immediately.

Nutrition:

Calories: 196,

Sodium: 21 mg,

Dietary Fibre: 1.4 g, Total Fat: 1.1 g,

Total Carbs: 1.6 g,

Protein: 1.5 g.

Strawberry Frozen Yogurt

Preparation Time: 10 minutes

Cooking Time: 15 minutes

Servings: 4

Ingredients:

15 ounces of plain yogurt

6 ounces of strawberries

Juice of 1 orange

1 tablespoon honey

Directions:

Place the strawberries and orange juice into a food processor or blender and blitz until smooth. Press the mixture through a sieve into a large bowl to remove seeds. Stir in the honey and yogurt. Transfer the mixture to an ice-cream maker and follow the manufacturer's instructions. Alternatively, pour the mixture into a container and place in the fridge for 1 hour. Use a fork to whisk it and break up ice crystals and freeze for 2 hours.

Nutrition:

Calories: 238,

Sodium: 33 mg,

Dietary Fibre: 1.4 g,

Total Fat: 1.8 g,

Total Carbs: 12.3 g,

Protein: 1.3 g.

Berry Soy Yogurt Parfait

Preparation Time: 2-4 minutes

Cooking Time: 0 minute

Servings: 1

Ingredients:

One carton vanilla cultured soy yoghurt

1/4 cup granola (gluten-free)

1 cup berries (you can take strawberries, blueberries, raspberries, blackberries)

Directions

Put half of the yogurt in a glass jar or serving dish.

On the top put half of the berries.

Then sprinkle with half of granola

Repeat layers.

Nutrition:

Calories: 244,

Sodium: 33 mg,

Dietary Fibre: 1.4 g,

Total Fat: 3.1 g,

Total Carbs: 11.3 g,

Protein: 1.4 g.

Orange & Celery Crush

Preparation Time: 10 minutes

Cooking Time: 0 minutes

Servings: 1

Ingredients:

1 carrot, peeled

Stalks of celery

1 orange, peeled

½ teaspoon matcha powder

Juice of 1 lime

Directions:

Place ingredients into a blender with enough water to cover them and blitz until smooth.

Nutrition:

Calories: 150,

Sodium: 31 mg,

Dietary Fibre: 1.2 g,

Total Fat: 2.1 g,

Total Carbs: 11.2 g,

Protein: 1.4 g.

Creamy Strawberry & Cherry Smoothie

Preparation Time: 10 minutes

Cooking Time: 15 minutes

Servings: 1

Ingredients:

3½ ounce. Strawberries

3.5 ounce of frozen pitted cherries

One tablespoon plain full-fat yogurt

6.5 ounce of unsweetened soya milk

Directions:

Place the ingredients into a blender then process until smooth. Serve and enjoy.

Nutrition:

Calories: 203,

Sodium: 23 mg, Dietary Fibre: 1.4 g,

Total Fat: 3.1 g, Total Carbs: 12.3 g,

Protein: 1.7 g.

Grapefruit & Celery Blast

Preparation Time: 10 minutes

Cooking Time: 15 minutes

Servings: 1

Ingredients:

1 grapefruit, peeled

stalks of celery

2-ounce kale

½ teaspoon matcha powder

Directions:

Place ingredients into a blender with water to cover them and blitz until smooth.

Nutrition:

Calories: 129,

Sodium: 24 mg,

Dietary Fibre: 1.4 g,

Total Fat: 2.1 g,

Total Carbs: 12.1 g,

Protein: 1.2 g.

Walnut & Spiced Apple Tonic

Preparation Time: 10 minutes

Cooking Time: 15 minutes

Servings: 1

Ingredients:

6 walnuts halves

1 apple, cored

1 banana

½ teaspoon matcha powder

½ teaspoon cinnamon

Pinch of ground nutmeg

Directions:

Place ingredients into a blender and add sufficient water to cover them. Blitz until smooth and creamy.

Nutrition:

Calories: 124, Sodium: 22 mg,

Dietary Fibre: 1.4 g,

Total Fat: 2.1 g, Total Carbs: 12.3 g,

Protein: 1.2 g.

Tropical Chocolate Delight

Preparation Time: 10 minutes

Cooking Time: 15 minutes

Servings: 1

Ingredients:

1 mango, peeled & de-stoned

ounce fresh pineapple, chopped

2 ounces of kale

1 ounce of rocket

1 tablespoon 100% cocoa powder or cacao nibs

1 ounce of coconut milk

Directions:

Place ingredients into a blender and blitz until smooth. You can add a little water if it seems too thick.

Nutrition:

Calories: 192, Sodium: 26 mg,

Dietary Fibre: 1.3 g, Total Fat: 4.1 g,

Total Carbs: 16.6 g, Protein: 1.6 g.

CHAPTER 28:

Appetizers Recipes

Basic Cauliflower Rice

Preparation Time: 5 Minutes

Cooking Time: 6 Minutes

Servings: 6 (1/2 cup)

Ingredients:

2 lb Raw,

Organic Cauliflower

Cheese Bag

Directions

Prepare the Cauliflower: Wash and trim away the stems and leaves.

Blend the Cauliflower: chop the cauliflower, so it's easier on your blender. Add into a blender with just enough water to cover. Pulse until your cauliflower resembles rice.

Strain the cauliflower through a cheese bag. You now have perfectly riced cauliflower ready to eat as is, or cook!

Nutrition

Calories 10 Fat 0g

Protein 1g

7 Minute Zoodles (Zucchini Noodles)

Preparation Time: 5 Minutes

Cooking Time: 2 Minutes

Servings: 4 (1 cup each)

Ingredients:

3 lbs Zucchini

Spiral Slicer

Olive Oil

Directions

Prepare the Zucchini: trim the ends away from your zucchini.

Using the instructions to your spiral slicer, slice the zucchini into noodles. Store, Or Cook: Simply heat a saucepan with olive oil over medium heat. Saute zoodles for 5 minutes, until tender!

Nutrition

Calories 21 Fat 0g

Protein 2g

Trout and Chili Nuts

Preparation Time: 10 minutes

Cooking time: 0 minutes

Servings: 3

Ingredients:

1.5kg of rainbow trout

300gr shelled walnuts

1 bunch of parsley

9 cloves of garlic

7 tablespoons of olive oil

2 fresh hot peppers

The juice of 2 lemons

Halls

Directions:

Clean and dry the trout, then place them in a baking tray.

Chop the walnuts, parsley and chili peppers, then mash the garlic cloves.

Mix the Ingredients by adding olive oil, lemon juice and a pinch of salt.

Stuff the trout with some of the sauce and use the rest to cover the fish.

Bake at 180° for 30/40 minutes.

Serve the trout hot or cold.

Nutrition:

Calories 226

Fat 5

Fiber 2

Carbs 7

Protein 8

Nut Granola & Smoothie Bowl

Preparation Time: 10 minutes

Cooking time: 40 minutes

Servings: 3

Ingredients:

6 cups Greek yogurt

4 tablespoon almond butter

A handful toasted walnuts

3 tablespoon unsweetened cocoa powder

4 teaspoon swerve brown sugar

2 cups nut granola for topping

Directions:

Combine the Greek yogurt, almond butter, walnuts, cocoa powder, and swerve brown sugar in a smoothie maker; puree in high-speed until smooth and well mixed.

Share the smoothie into four breakfast bowls, top with a half cup of granola each, and serve.

Nutrition:

Kcal 361,

Fat 31.2g,

Net Carbs 2g,

Protein 13g

Bacon and Egg Quesadillas

Preparation Time: 10 minutes

Cooking time: 30 minutes

Servings: 3

Ingredients:

8 low carb tortilla shells

6 eggs - 1 cup of water

3 tablespoon butter

1 ½ cups grated cheddar cheese

1 ½ cups grated Swiss cheese

5 bacon slices - 1 medium onion, thinly sliced

1 tablespoon chopped parsley

Directions

Bring the eggs to a boil in water over medium heat for 10 minutes. Transfer the eggs to an ice water bath, peel the shells, and chop them; set aside.

Meanwhile, as the eggs cook, fry the bacon in a skillet over medium heat for 4 minutes until crispy. Remove and chop. Plate and set aside too.

Fetch out 2/3 of the bacon fat and sauté the onions in the remaining grease over medium heat for 2 minutes; set aside. Melt 1 tablespoon of butter in a skillet over medium heat. Lay one tortilla in a skillet; sprinkle with some Swiss cheese. Add some chopped eggs and bacon over the cheese, top with onion, and sprinkle with some cheddar cheese. Cover with another tortilla shell. Cook for 45 seconds, then carefully flip the quesadilla, and cook the other side too for 45 seconds. Remove to a plate and repeat the cooking process using the remaining tortilla shells.

Garnish with parsley and serve warm.

Nutrition:

Kcal 449, Fat 48.7g, Net Carbs 6.8g,

Protein 29.1g

Avocado and Kale Eggs

Preparation Time: 10 minutes

Cooking time: 30 minutes

Servings: 3

Ingredients:

1 teaspoon ghee

1 red onion, sliced

4 oz chorizo, cut into thin rounds

1 cup chopped kale

1 ripe avocado, pitted, peeled, chopped

4 eggs

Salt and black pepper to season

Directions:

Preheat oven to 370ºF.

Melt ghee in a cast iron pan over medium heat and sauté the onion for 2 minutes. Add the chorizo and cook for 2 minutes more, flipping once.

Introduce the kale in batches with a splash of water to wilt, season lightly with salt, stir and cook for 3 minutes. Mix in the avocado and turn the heat off.

Create four holes in the mixture, crack the eggs into each hole, sprinkle with salt and black pepper, and slide the pan into the preheated oven to bake for 6 minutes until the egg whites are set or firm and yolks still runny. Season to taste with salt and pepper, and serve right away with low carb toasts.

Nutrition:

Kcal 274,

Fat 23g,

Net Carbs 4g,

Protein 13g

Bacon and Cheese Frittata

Preparation Time: 10 minutes

Cooking time: 20 minutes

Servings: 3

Ingredients:

10 slices bacon

10 fresh eggs

3 tablespoon butter, melted

½ cup almond milk

Salt and black pepper to taste

1 ½ cups cheddar cheese, shredded

¼ cup chopped green onions

Directions:

Preheat the oven to 400°F and grease a baking dish with cooking spray. Cook the bacon in a skillet over medium heat for 6 minutes. Once crispy, remove from the skillet to paper towels and discard grease. Chop into small pieces. Whisk the eggs, butter, milk, salt, and black pepper. Mix in the bacon and pour the mixture into the baking dish.

Sprinkle with cheddar cheese and green onions, and bake in the oven for 10 minutes or until the eggs are thoroughly cooked. Remove and cool the frittata for 3 minutes, slice into wedges, and serve warm with a dollop of Greek yogurt.

Nutrition:

Kcal 325,

Fat 28g,

Net Carbs 2g,

Protein 15g

Spicy Egg Muffins with Bacon & Cheese

Preparation Time: 10 minutes

Cooking time: 20 minutes

Servings: 3

Ingredients:

12 eggs

¼ cup of coconut milk

Salt and black pepper to taste

1 cup grated cheddar cheese

12 slices bacon

4 jalapeño peppers, seeded and minced

Directions:

Preheat oven to 370°F.

Crack the eggs into a bowl and whisk with coconut milk until combined. Season with salt and pepper, and evenly stir in the cheddar cheese.

Line each hole of a muffin tin with a slice of bacon and fill each with the egg mixture two-thirds way up. Top with the jalapeno peppers and bake in the oven for 18 to 20 minutes or until puffed and golden. Remove, allow cooling for a few minutes, and serve with arugula salad.

Nutrition:

Kcal 302,

Fat 23.7g,

Net Carbs 3.2g,

Protein 20g

Ham & Egg Broccoli Bake

Preparation Time: 10 minutes

Cooking time: 25 minutes

Servings: 3

Ingredients:

2 heads broccoli, cut into small florets

2 red bell peppers, seeded and chopped

¼ cup chopped ham - 2 teaspoon ghee

1 teaspoon dried oregano + extra to garnish

Salt and black pepper to taste - 8 fresh eggs

Directions

Preheat oven to 425°F. Melt the ghee in a frying pan over medium heat; brown the ham, frequently stirring, about 3 minutes. Arrange the broccoli, bell peppers, and ham on a foil-lined baking sheet in a single layer, toss to combine; season with salt, oregano, and black pepper. Bake for 10 minutes until the vegetables have softened. Remove, create eight indentations with a spoon, and crack an egg into each. Return to the oven and continue to bake for an additional 5 to 7 minutes until the egg whites are firm. Season with salt, black pepper, and extra oregano, share the bake into four plates and serve with strawberry lemonade (optional).

Nutrition: Kcal 344, Fat 28g, Net Carbs 4.2g, Protein 11g

Secret Guacamole

Preparation Time: 5 Minutes

Cooking Time 0

Servings: 8 (¼ cup of guacamole)

Ingredients:

4 Medium Avocados

1/2 cup fresh salsa

2 tbsp chopped cilantro

1 tbsp lime

1 tsp minced garlic

1 tbsp minced red onions

¼ tsp chipotle powder

fine sea salt

Directions

Prepare the guacamole:

Mash avocados with a fork in a bowl.

Add remaining ingredients. Stir until evenly mixed.

Nutrition

Calories 51 Fat 4g

Protein 1g

CHAPTER 29:

Salad Recipes

Tomato & Mozzarella Salad

Preparation time: 15 minutes

Cooking time: 0 minutes

Servings: 8

Ingredients:

4 cups cherry tomatoes, halved

1½ pounds mozzarella cheese, cubed

¼ cup fresh basil leaves, chopped

¼ cup olive oil

2 tablespoons fresh lemon juice

1 teaspoon fresh oregano, minced

1 teaspoon fresh parsley, minced

2–4 drops liquid stevia

Salt and ground black pepper, as required

Directions:

In a salad bowl, mix tomatoes, mozzarella, and basil. In a small bowl, add remaining ingredients and beat until well combined. Place dressing over salad and toss to coat well. Serve immediately.

Nutrition:

Calories 87 Net Carbs 2.7 g

Total Fat 7.5 g Saturated Fat 1.5 g

Cholesterol 3 mg Sodium 57 mg

Total Carbs 3.9 g Fiber 1.2 g

Sugar 2.5 g Protein 2.4 g

Cucumber & Tomato Salad

Preparation time: 15 minutes

Cooking time: 0 minutes

Servings: 8

Ingredients: Salad

3 large English cucumbers, thinly sliced

2 cups tomatoes, chopped - 6 cups lettuce, torn

Dressing - 4 tablespoons olive oil

2 tablespoons balsamic vinegar

1 tablespoon fresh lemon juice

Salt and ground black pepper, as required

Directions:

For the salad: In a large bowl, add the cucumbers, onion, cucumbers, and mix.

For the dressing: In a small bowl, add all the ingredients and beat until well combined.

Place the dressing over the salad and toss to coat well. Serve immediately.

Nutrition:

Calories 86 Net Carbs 0 g Total Fat 7.3 g

Saturated Fat 1 g Cholesterol 0 mg

Sodium 27 mg Total Carbs 5.1 g

Fiber 1.4 g Sugar 2.8 g

Protein 1.1 g

Chicken & Strawberry Salad

Preparation time: 20 minutes

Cooking time: 16 minutes

Servings: 8

Ingredients:

2 pounds grass-fed boneless skinless chicken breasts

½ cup olive oil

¼ cup fresh lemon juice

2 tablespoons granulated erythritol

1 garlic clove, minced

Salt and ground black pepper, as required

4 cups fresh strawberries

8 cups fresh spinach, torn

Directions:

For the marinade: in a large bowl, add oil, lemon juice, erythritol, garlic, salt, and black pepper, and beat until well combined.

In a large resealable plastic bag, place the chicken and ¾ cup of marinade.

Seal bag and shake to coat well.

Refrigerate overnight.

Cover the bowl of remaining marinade and refrigerate before serving.

Preheat the grill to medium heat. Grease the grill grate.

Remove the chicken from the bag and discard the marinade.

Place the chicken onto grill grate and grill, covered for about 5–8 minutes per side.

Remove chicken from grill and cut into bite-sized pieces.

In a large bowl, add the chicken pieces, strawberries, and spinach, and mix.

Place the reserved marinade and toss to coat.

Serve immediately.

Nutrition:

Calories 356

Net Carbs 4 g

Total Fat 21.4 g

Saturated Fat 4 g

Cholesterol 101 mg

Sodium 143 mg

Total Carbs 6.1 g

Fiber 2.1 g

Sugar 3.8 g

Protein 34.2 g

Salmon Salad

Preparation time: 15 minutes

Cooking time: 0 minutes

Servings: 8

Ingredients:

12 hard-boiled organic eggs, peeled and cubed

1 pound smoked salmon

3 celery stalks, chopped

1 yellow onion, chopped

4 tablespoons fresh dill, chopped

2 cups mayonnaise

Salt and ground black pepper, as required

8 cups fresh lettuce leaves

Directions:

In a large serving bowl, add all the ingredients (except the lettuce leaves) and gently stir to combine.

Cover and refrigerate to chill before serving.

Divide the lettuce onto serving plates and top with the salmon salad.

Serve immediately.

Nutrition:

Calories 539 Net Carbs 3.5 g

Total Fat 49.2 g Saturated Fat 8.6 g

Cholesterol 279 mg Sodium 1618 mg

Total Carbs 4.5 g Fiber 1 g

Sugar 1.7 g Protein 19.4 g

Shrimp Salad

Preparation time: 15 minutes

Cooking time: 6 minutes

Servings: 6

Ingredients:

1 tablespoon unsalted butter

1 garlic clove, crushed and divided

2 tablespoons fresh rosemary, chopped

1 pound shrimp, peeled and deveined

Salt and ground black pepper, as required

4 cups fresh arugula

2 cups lettuce, torn

2 tablespoons olive oil

2 tablespoons fresh lime juice

Directions:

In a large wok, melt the butter over medium heat and sauté 1 garlic clove for about 1 minute.

Add the shrimp with salt and black pepper and cook for about 4–5 minutes.

Remove from the heat and set aside to cool.

Ina large bowl, add the shrimp, arugula, oil, lime juice, salt, and black pepper, and gently toss to coat.

Serve immediately.

Nutrition:

Calories 157

Net Carbs 2.3 g

Total Fat 8.2 g

Saturated Fat 2.4 g

Cholesterol 164 mg

Sodium 230 mg

Total Carbs 3.1 g

Fiber 0.8 g

Sugar 0.5 g

Protein 17.7 g

CHAPTER 30:

Bread Recipes

Keto Breakfast Bread

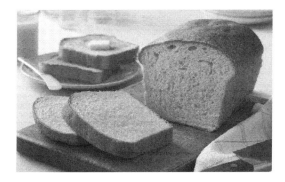

Preparation Time: 15 minutes

Cooking Time: 40 minutes

Servings: 16 slices

Ingredients:

½ tsp. Xanthan gum

½ tsp. salt

2 tbsp. coconut oil

½ cup butter, melted

1 tsp. baking powder

2 cups of almond flour

7 eggs

Directions:

Preheat the oven to 355F.

Beat eggs in a bowl on high for 2 minutes.

Add coconut oil and butter to the eggs and continue to beat.

Line a loaf pan with baking paper and pour the beaten eggs.

Pour in the rest of the Ingredients and mix until it becomes thick.

Bake until a toothpick comes out dry, about 40 to 45 minutes.

Nutrition:

Calories: 234

Fat: 23g

Carb: 1g

Protein: 7g

Pumpkin Bread

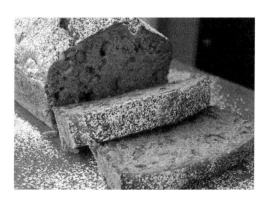

Preparation Time: 15 minutes

Cooking Time: 1 hour

Servings: 8

Ingredients:

3 tbsp. walnuts, chopped

3 tbsp. pumpkin seeds plus extra for topping

2 eggs

¼ cup no-sugar-added apple sauce

2 tbsp. Coconut oil

¾ cup pumpkin puree

½ tbsp. butter

1 tbsp. Pumpkin pie spice

½ tbsp. baking powder

½ tsp. salt

1 tbsp. psyllium husk powder

¼ cup flaxseed

½ cup almond flour

½ cup coconut flour

Directions:

Preheat the oven to 400F and grease a baking tray with butter.

Combine all the dry Ingredients in a bowl except pumpkin seeds.

Whisk together apple sauce, eggs, pumpkin puree, and oil in another bowl.

Combine the dry mixture with the egg mixture.

Transfer the mixture to a baking tray and sprinkle with pumpkin seeds.

Place the tray on the lower rack of the oven and bake for 1 hour.

Cool, slice, and serve.

Nutrition:

Calories: 194

Fat: 13.8g

Carb: 4.6g

Protein: 6.3g

Tasty Psyllium Husk Bread

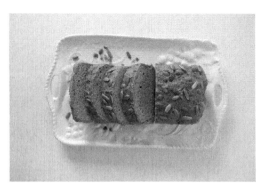

Preparation Time: 5 minutes

Cooking Time: 55 minutes

Servings: 15

Ingredients:

6 tbsp. whole psyllium husks (finely ground)

1 cup coconut flour - 8 egg whites

¾ tsp. sea salt

½ cup avocado oil

2 large eggs

1 ½ tsp. baking soda

¼ cup melted coconut oil

¾ cup of warm water

Directions:

Preheat the oven to 350F. Prepare a baking pan with parchment paper. Add every ingredient into a food processor and process until combined. Add batter into the prepared baking pan and spread until even at the top. Transfer baking pan into the preheated oven and bake for 45 to 55 minutes, or until an inserted toothpick comes out clean and bread edges are browned. Remove bread from the oven and cool for 15 minutes. Serve.

Nutrition:

Calories: 127 Fat: 13.3g Carb: 6g

Protein: 3g

Garlic Almond Bread

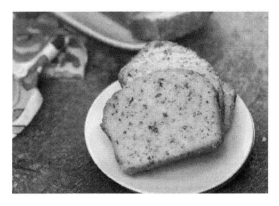

Preparation Time: 15 minutes

Cooking Time: 25 minutes

Servings: 8

Ingredients:

1 cup almond flour

3 eggs

3 tbsp. butter

¼ cup sour cream

1 cup cheddar cheese, shredded

½ tbsp. Baking powder

½ tbsp. Garlic, minced

¼ tsp. salt

2 tbsp. parsley, chopped

Directions:

Preheat the oven to 350F. Grease a round baking dish.

Combine butter, eggs, and sour cream in a bowl and whisk.

Combine cheddar cheese, almond flour, baking powder, minced garlic, and salt in another bowl and mix well.

Combine flour mixture with egg mixture and let the Ingredients integrate.

Transfer the batter into the baking dish and sprinkle with parsley.

Place in the oven and bake for 25 minutes.

Cool, slice, and serve.

Nutrition:

Calories: 220

Fat: 18.8g

Carb: 4.3g

Protein: 8.9g

Keto Cloud Bread

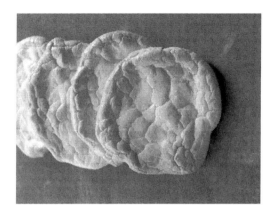

Preparation Time: 10 minutes

Cooking Time: 20 minutes

Servings: 12

Ingredients:

3 tbsp. cream cheese

3 eggs

½ tsp. Sea salt

¼ tsp. Baking powder

¼ tsp. pepper

Directions:

Preheat oven to 350F.

Add egg yolks and cream cheese into a bowl and mix with a hand mixer.

In another bowl, add egg whites, pepper, salt and baking powder and mix for 5 minutes or until stiff peaks form.

Add the egg yolk mixture and egg white mixture together until mixed well.

Transfer mixture into a loaf pan and place it into the prepared oven.

Bake for 15 to 18 minutes, or until lightly golden.

Nutrition:

Calories: 28

Fat: 2g

Carb: 0 g

Protein: 2g

Almond Cinnamon Bread

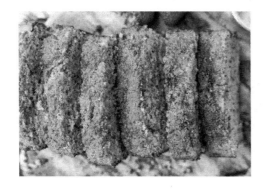

Preparation Time: 10 minutes

Cooking Time: 30 minutes

Servings: 9

Ingredients:

2 cups almond flour

2 tbsp. Coconut flour

½ tsp. sea salt

1 tsp. Baking soda

¼ cup flax seed meal.

Five eggs plus 1 egg white, whisked

1 ½ tsp. juiced lime

2 tbsp. no-sugar-added maple syrup

3 tbsp. butter, divided and melted

1 tbsp. cinnamon plus extra for topping

Directions:

Preheat the oven to 350F and line a loaf pan with parchment paper.

In a bowl, combine the almond flour, coconut flour, baking soda, salt, ½ tbsp. Cinnamon and flaxseed meal together.

In another bowl, add in the egg white and eggs and whisk together. Add in the maple syrup, butter, vinegar, and combine.

Pour the flour mixture into the egg mixture then mix to combine.

Transfer into the lined loaf pan.

Bake at 350F for 30 to 35 minutes. Remove.

Combine the remaining cinnamon and melted butter together then use it to rub the baked bread.

Cool, slice, and serve.

Nutrition:

Calories: 221

Fat: 15.4g

Carb: 10.7g

Protein: 9.3g

Fluffy Paleo Bread

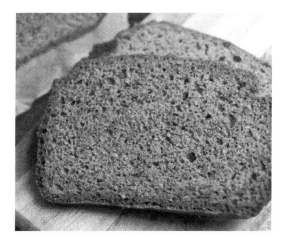

Preparation Time: 10 minutes

Cooking Time: 40 minutes

Servings: 15

Ingredients:

1 ¼ cup almond flour

5 eggs

1 tsp. lemon juice

1/3 cup avocado oil

1 dash black pepper

½ tsp. sea salt

3 to 4 tbsp. tapioca flour

1 to 2 tsp. poppy seed

¼ cup ground flaxseed

½ tsp. baking soda

Top with

Poppy seeds

Pumpkin seeds

Directions:

Preheat the oven to 350F.

Line a baking pan with parchment paper and set aside.

In a bowl, add eggs, avocado oil, and lemon juice and whisk until combined.

In another bowl, add tapioca flour, almond flour, baking soda, flaxseed, black pepper and poppy seed. Mix.

Add the lemon juice mixture into the flour mixture and mix well.

Add the batter into the loaf pan. Top with extra pumpkin seeds and poppy seeds. Cover loaf pan and transfer into the prepared oven. Bake for 20 minutes. Remove cover and bake until an inserted knife comes out clean after about 15 to 20 minutes. Remove from oven and cool. Slice and serve.

Nutrition:

Calories: 149 Fat: 12.9g Carb: 4.4g Protein: 5g

Low-Carb Holiday Bread

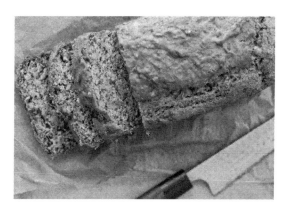

Preparation Time: 25 minutes

Cooking Time: 1 hour

Servings: 12

Ingredients:

1 cup almond flour

¼ cup coconut flour

3 tbsp. sesame seeds

3 tbsp. flaxseed

2 tbsp. Psyllium husk powder

½ tbsp. Baking powder

½ tsp. salt

Three eggs

½ cup sour cream

¼ cup cream cheese

1 tbsp. Cloves, ground

½ tbsp. Bitter orange peel, ground

½ tbsp. fennel seeds

1 tsp. anise seeds

1 tsp. cardamom, ground

Directions:

Preheat the oven to 400F and lightly grease a loaf pan.

Mix all the dry ingredients in a bowl.

Whisk together eggs, sour cream, and cream cheese in another bowl.

Combine the dry mixture with the egg mixture and stir well.

Transfer the mixture to the loaf pan and place in the oven.

Slice and serve.

Nutrition:

Calories: 85

Fat: 6.6g

Carb: 4g

Protein: 2.9g

Sandwich Bread

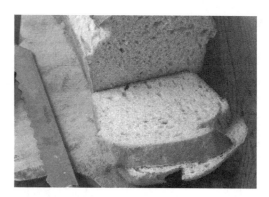

Preparation Time: 10 minutes

Cooking Time: 45 minutes

Servings: 8

Ingredients:

½ cup coconut flour sifted

¼ cup almond flour, sifted

6 eggs, whites and yolks separated

½ cup coconut oil

¼ tsp. salt

3 tbsp. water

1 tbsp. Apple cider vinegar

½ tsp. baking powder

Directions:

Preheat the oven to 350F.

Grease an (8 ½ by 4-inch) loaf pan with oil.

Place a piece of parchment paper on the bottom of the pan.

Cream coconut oil in a food processor and add egg yolks at a time.

Pulse to combine coconut oil and yolks.

Add sifted coconut and almond flour, baking powder, apple cider vinegar, salt, and water to a food processor and pulse until combined.

Take a mixing bowl and beat egg whites.

Fold in coconut flour. Mix into egg whites and mix.

Pour the batter into prepared loaf pan and bake for 40 to 45 minutes. Cover it with aluminum foil about halfway through.

Let it cool and slice.

Enjoy.

Nutrition:

Calories: 146 Fat: 11g Carb: 7g Protein: 5g

No Corn Cornbread

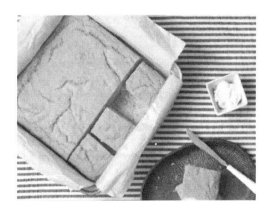

Preparation Time: 10 minutes

Cooking Time: 20 minutes

Servings: 8

Ingredients:

½ cup almond flour

¼ cup coconut flour

¼ tsp. salt

¼ tsp. baking soda

3 eggs

¼ cup unsalted butter

2 tbsp. low-carb sweetener

½ cup of coconut milk

Directions:

Preheat the oven to 325F. Line a baking pan.

Mix all the dry ingredients in a bowl.

Add all the wet ingredients to the dry ones and blend well.

Pour the batter into the baking pan and bake for 20 minutes.

Cool, slice, and serve.

Nutrition:

Calories: 65 Fat: 6g Carb: 2g Protein: 2g

Double Chocolate Zucchini Bread

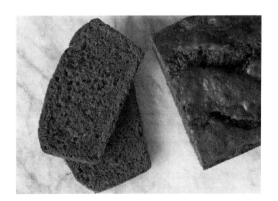

Preparation Time: 10 minutes

Cooking Time: 55 minutes

Servings: 12

Ingredients:

½ cup coconut flour

½ cup of chocolate chips (sugar-free)

2 cups zucchini (shredded)

1 tsp. vanilla

Four large eggs

¼ cup coconut oil, melted

¼ tsp. salt

1 tsp. baking powder

1 tsp. baking soda

½ tsp. ground cinnamon

½ cup low carb sweetener

½ cup cocoa powder (unsweetened)

Directions:

In a bowl, combine coconut flour, salt, baking powder, cinnamon, sweetener, baking soda, and cocoa. Blend in the vanilla, coconut oil, and eggs. Mix well. Fold in the chocolate chips and zucchini. Line a loaf pan (9 x 5) with parchment paper and pour the mixture in it. Bake at 350F for 45 to 55 minutes. Remove from the oven and cool. Serve.

Nutrition:

Calories: 124 Fat: 10g Carb: 7g Protein: 4g

Keto Blueberry Bread

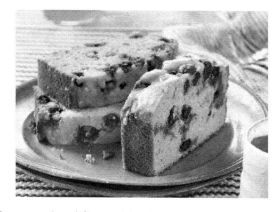

Preparation Time: 15 minutes

Cooking Time: 1 hour 10 minutes

Servings: 12

Ingredients:

10 tbsp. coconut flour

1 ½ tsp. Baking powder

½ tsp. salt

2 tbsp. heavy whipping cream

1 ½ tsp. vanilla

2/3 cup Monkfruit classic

2 tbsp. Sour cream

½ tsp. cinnamon

¾ cup fresh blueberries

9 tbsp. melted butter

6 eggs

For the icing

¼ tsp. lemon zest

1 tbsp. heavy whipping cream

dash of vanilla

1 tsp. butter (melted)

2 tbsp. Monkfruit powdered

Directions:

Line a regular loaf pan with parchment paper and preheat oven to 350F.

Melt butter.

Beat eggs, cinnamon, baking powder, salt, vanilla, whipping cream, sour cream, and Monkfruit until combined.

Add melted butter and mix well.

Add coconut flour and mix well.

Add a small amount of batter in the loaf pan and sprinkle with a couple of blueberries. Then spread more batter and sprinkle blueberries on top. Repeat to finish the batter and blueberries.

Bake for 65 to 75 minutes. Cool.

For the icing, combine all ingredients and whisk.

Drizzle over warm bread and serve.

Nutrition:

Calories: 155 Fat: 13g Carb: 4g Protein: 3g

CHAPTER 31:

Condiments, Sauces, & Spreads Recipes

Curry Powder

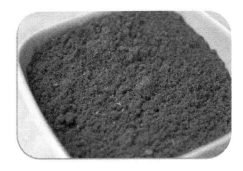

Preparation time: 10 minutes

Cooking time: 10 minutes

Servings: 20

Ingredients:

¼ cup coriander seeds

2 tablespoons mustard seeds

2 tablespoons cumin seeds

2 tablespoons anise seeds

1 tablespoon whole allspice berries

1 tablespoon fenugreek seeds

5 tablespoons ground turmeric

Directions:

In a large nonstick frying pan, place all the spices except turmeric over medium heat and cook for about 9–10 minutes or until toasted completely, stirring continuously.

Remove the frying pan from heat and set aside to cool.

In a spice grinder, add the toasted spices and turmeric, and grind until a subtle powder forms.

Transfer into an airtight jar to preserve.

Nutrition:

Calories 18

Net Carbs 1.8 g

Total Fat 0.8 g

Saturated Fat 0.1 g

Cholesterol 0 mg

Sodium 3 mg

Total Carbs 2.7 g

Fiber 0.9 g

Sugar 0.1 g

Protein 0.8 g

Poultry Seasoning

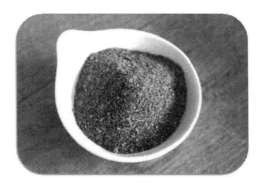

Preparation time: 5 minutes

Cooking time: 5 minutes

Servings: 10

Ingredients:

2 teaspoons dried sage, crushed finely

1 teaspoon dried marjoram, crushed finely

¾ teaspoon dried rosemary, crushed finely

1½ teaspoons dried thyme, crushed finely

½ teaspoon ground nutmeg

½ teaspoon ground black pepper

Directions:

Add all the ingredients in a bowl and stir to combine.

Transfer into an airtight jar to preserve.

Nutrition:

Calories 2

Net Carbs 0.2 g

Total Fat 0.1g Saturated Fat 0.1 g

Cholesterol 0 mg

Sodium 0 mg   Total Carbs 0.4 g

Fiber 0.2 g

Sugar 0 g

Protein 0.1 g

BBQ Sauce

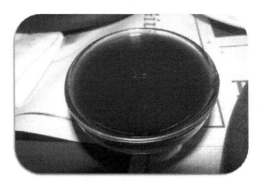

Preparation time: 15 minutes

Cooking time: 20 minutes

Servings: 20

Ingredients:

2½ (6-ounces) cans sugar-free tomato paste

½ cup organic apple cider vinegar

1/3 cup powdered erythritol

2 tablespoons Worcestershire sauce

1 tablespoon liquid smoke

2 teaspoons smoked paprika

1 teaspoon garlic powder

½ teaspoon onion powder

Salt, as required - ¼ teaspoon red chili powder

¼ teaspoon cayenne pepper

1½ cups water

Directions:

Add all the ingredients (except the water) in a pan and beat until well combined.

Add 1 cup of water and beat until combined.

Add the remaining water and beat until well combined.

Place the pan over medium-high heat and bring to a gentle boil.

Adjust the heat to medium-low and simmer, uncovered for about 20 minutes, stirring frequently.

Remove the pan of sauce from the heat and set aside to cool slightly before serving.

You can preserve this sauce in refrigerator by placing it into an airtight container.

Nutrition:

Calories 22 Net Carbs 3.7 g

Total Fat 0.1 g Saturated Fat 0 g

Cholesterol 0 mg

Sodium 46 mg Total Carbs 4.7 g

Fiber 1 g Sugar 3 g Protein 1 g

Ketchup

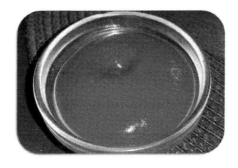

Preparation time: 10 minutes

Cooking time: 30 minutes

Servings: 12

Ingredients:

6 ounces sugar-free tomato paste

1 cup of water

¼ cup powdered erythritol

3 tablespoons balsamic vinegar

½ teaspoon garlic powder

½ teaspoon onion powder

¼ teaspoon paprika

1/8 teaspoon ground cloves

1/8 teaspoon mustard powder

Salt, as required

Directions:

Add all ingredients in a small pan and beat until smooth.

Now, place the pan over medium heat and bring to a gentle simmer, stirring continuously.

Adjust the heat to low and simmer, covered for about 30 minutes or until desired thickness, stirring occasionally.

Remove the pan from heat and with an immersion blender, blend until smooth.

Now, set aside to cool completely before serving.

You can preserve this ketchup in the refrigerator by placing it in an airtight container.

Nutrition:

Calories 13

Net Carbs 2.3 g

Total Fat 0.1 g

Saturated Fat 0 g

Cholesterol 0 mg

Sodium 26 mg

Total Carbs 2.9 g

Fiber 0.6 g

Sugar 1.8 g

Protein 0.7 g

Cranberry Sauce

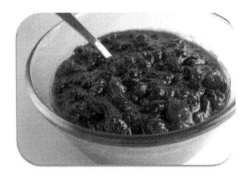

Preparation time: 10 minutes

Cooking time: 15 minutes

Servings: 6

Ingredients:

12 ounces fresh cranberries

1 cup powdered erythritol

¾ cup of water

1 teaspoon fresh lemon zest, grated

½ teaspoon organic vanilla extract

Directions:

Place the cranberries, water, erythritol, and lemon zest in a medium pan and mix well. Place the pan over medium heat and bring to a boil. Adjust the heat to low and simmer for about 12–15 minutes, stirring frequently. Remove the pan from heat and mix in the vanilla extract. Set aside at room temperature to cool completely. Transfer the sauce into a bowl and refrigerate to chill before serving.

Nutrition:

Calories 32 Net Carbs 3.2 g

Total Fat 0 g Saturated Fat 0 g

Cholesterol 0 mg Sodium 1 mg

Total Carbs 5.3 g Fiber 2.1 g

Sugar 2.1 g Protein 0 g

Yogurt Tzatziki

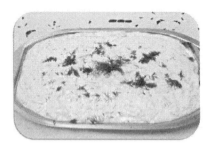

Preparation time: 10 minutes

Cooking time: 0 minutes

Servings: 12

Ingredients:

1 large English cucumber, peeled and grated

Salt, as required - 2 cups plain Greek yogurt

1 tablespoon fresh lemon juice

4 garlic cloves, minced

1 tablespoon fresh mint leaves, chopped

2 tablespoons fresh dill, chopped

Pinch of cayenne pepper

Ground black pepper, as required

Directions:

Arrange a colander in the sink. Place the cucumber into the colander and sprinkle with salt. Let it drain for about 10–15 minutes. With your hands, squeeze the cucumber well. Place the cucumber and remaining ingredients in a large bowl and stir to combine. Cover the bowl and place in the refrigerator to chill for at least 4–8 hours before serving.

Nutrition:

Calories 36 Net Carbs 4.2 g   Total Fat 0.6 g

Saturated Fat 0.4 g   Cholesterol 2 mg

Sodium 42 mg Total Carbs 4.5 g

Fiber 0.3 g Sugar 3.3 g   Protein 2.7 g

Conclusion

The ketogenic diet is one that has many important aspects and information that you need to know as someone who wants to try this diet. It is important to remember the warning that we have given you at the beginning of the book that this is not a diet that is safe and that doctors recommend you don't try it, or if you are going to attempt it remember that you shouldn't do so for longer than six months and even then never without the constant supervision of a doctor or at the very least a doctor knowing that you're doing this. You following their guidelines and words exactly so that they can make sure that you are safe.

The ketogenic diet is a diet that believes that by minimizing your carbs, you will, while maximizing the good fat in your system and making sure that you're getting the protein you need, that you will be happier and healthier. In this book, we give you the information to know what this diet is all about, as well as describing the different types and areas that this diet will offer. Most people assume that there is only one way to do this. While there is one thing that the additional options share, there are four different options you can choose from. Each one has it's unique benefits, and you should know about each type to learn what would be best for your body, which is why we have described them in the book for you to have the best information possible when you begin this diet for yourself.

Another big thing about this diet is that many people don't understand the importance of exercise with this diet. The best way to become healthier is to do three things for yourself. Get the right amount of sleep, eat healthily, and make sure that you get the proper amount of exercise as well for your body to work at an optimum level. As such, we explain the exercises that are the best to go with your diet to make sure that you are getting the most out of it.

For women who are on the go and have a busy lifestyle, we have provided recipes for a thirty-day meal plan so that you can make food quickly and have a great meal for your lifestyle. They also have enough servings for you to have leftovers so that you don't have to worry about preparing in the morning. Instead, you can simply pack it up and take it with you wherever you go. This works out so much easier for so many people because they don't have to cook in the morning, and it saves a busy person a lot of time.

We also provide helpful ideas on how you can use these recipes for meals to make sure that you see how the numbers will affect you and make an impact on your day. A great example that we have explained is if you have a big breakfast that is full of the protein you need, for example, thirty grams, you've got to take note of this and be aware because if you eat too much for your dinner or another meal, you will throw your numbers out of where they are supposed to be. For those that have more time on their hands, we offer a thirty-day meal plan for you as well with all-new recipes to enjoy and tips and tricks for making them work for you in the best way.

With all of this information at your fingertips, you will be able to enjoy this diet and use it to your advantage. Another benefit that we offer? We explain routines that you can do for yourself to make this diet last longer for you and to benefit your body better as a result. Routines are very important and can be a big help to your body but also your spirit and your mind. This will help you utilize the diet better, and you will be able to improve with it as well as have it become easier for you to handle.

As many people are using this diet to their benefit, knowing your food is one of the biggest parts of this, and it becomes easier once you begin to use this in your daily life. One of the best things you can do is pay attention to the food that your eating and how it affects your body and mind. You will notice that this diet can make you sick, which isn't a good thing, and it's one of the things the doctors warn against. For this reason, it's very important to pay attention to what your eating and how your feeling at the same time. Another warning that we have said you need to pay attention to is that you will need to make sure that your ketogenic 'flu' isn't the result of something more serious. As people are being told that this is normal, this book has brought you the knowledge you need to be able to tell you why it's not.

This book has given you all the information you need to do this diet properly and to do it well. It's important to understand what you're getting into when you go into this diet. This book will give you valuable information that you can use to your benefit and so you can avoid the problems that can come with this diet. You want to stay healthy and make sure that your body can do what it needs to. As with anything, we have put a strong emphasis on the fact that if anything feels wrong or unnatural, you will need to see a doctor make sure that you are safe and that your body can handle this diet. Use the knowledge in this book to have amazing recipes and learn directions amazing meals for yourself.

Resources

Balduzzi, A. (n.d.). Is the Ketogenic Diet a Good Choice for Women Over 50? Retrieved from https://fitmotherproject.com/keto-for-women-over-50/

Easy Low Carb Egg Salad and Day One Back on Keto. (July 12). Retrieved from https://www.ibreatheimhungry.com/easy-low-carb-egg-salad-day-one-back-keto/

Keto Blueberry Yogurt Muffins. (2019). Retrieved from https://alldayidreamaboutfood.com/keto-blueberry-muffins/

Keto Pecan Crescent Cookies. (2018). Retrieved from https://alldayidreamaboutfood.com/pecan-crescents-and-a-pampered-chef-giveaway/

Raman, R. (2019). 7 Simple and Delicious Keto Salads. Retrieved, from https://www.healthline.com/nutrition/keto-salads

Rege, L. (2019). These Keto Chocolate Chip Cookies Are Gluten-Free, Sugar-Free, And Taste AMAZING. Retrieved from https://www.delish.com/cooking/recipe-ideas/a25752891/keto-chocolate-chip-cookie-recipe/

https://www.researchgate.net/publication/317858823_Fasting_as_possible_complementary_approach_for_polycystic_ovary_syndrome_Hope_or_hype

https://www.researchgate.net/publication/337691456_Intermittent_fasting_for_the_prevention_of_cardiovascular_disease

https://www.researchgate.net/publication/318498553_Metabolic_Effects_of_Intermittent_Fasting

Made in the USA
Middletown, DE
23 October 2020